THE
SCLERODERMA
BOOK

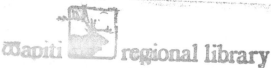
● ● ● ● ● ● ● ● ● ● ● ● ● ● ●

THE
SCLERODERMA
BOOK

*A Guide for Patients
and Families*

● ● ● ● ● ● ● ● ● ● ● ●

Maureen D. Mayes, M.D.

New York   Oxford
OXFORD UNIVERSITY PRESS
1999

Oxford University Press

Oxford   New York
Athens   Auckland   Bangkok   Bogotá   Buenos Aires
Calcutta   Cape Town   Chennai   Dar es Salaam   Delhi   Florence
Hong Kong   Istanbul   Karachi   Kuala Lumpur   Madrid
Melbourne   Mexico City   Mumbai   Nairobi   Paris
São Paulo   Singapore   Taipei   Tokyo   Toronto   Warsaw

and associated companies in
Berlin   Ibadan

Published by Oxford University Press, Inc.,
198 Madison Avenue, New York, New York 10016

Library of Congress Cataloging-in-Publication Data
Mayes, Maureen D.
The scleroderma book : a guide for patients
and families / Maureen D. Mayes.
p. cm.   Includes index.
ISBN 0-19-511507-4
1. Scleroderma (disease)—popular works.   I. Title.
RL451.M39   1999
616.5'44—dc21   98-54669

3 5 7 9 8 6 4 2

Printed in the United States of America
on acid-free paper

This book is dedicated to my family:
my husband, Chuck, and my sons, David and Ted,
without whose support I could not have written it.

This book is also dedicated to my patients,
who provided the source of inspiration and from
whom I have learned a great deal.

CONTENTS
✳ ✳ ✳

PREFACE

* * *

$\mathbf{T}$his book is meant for patients and their families who would like to know more about the disease of scleroderma. I do not expect people to read it from cover to cover, but suggest that individuals read the chapters that seem most relevant to them and to keep it as a reference when more questions or new issues arise.

Many patients find it difficult to talk about their disease to their friends and family members, since they themselves lack a medical background and are afraid of getting the facts "wrong." Others cannot bring themselves to talk to loved ones about the possible complications that could develop. On the other side of this communication gap are family members who feel left out of the picture, not even knowing what questions to ask. I hope that by sharing the information in this book, people find it easier to talk about these issues.

I also hope that this book can help to explain some of the

medical terminology and make the entire process more understandable and less intimidating. Modern medicine is a complex system of specialists and procedures with a peculiar vocabulary all its own.

As I sat down to write these chapters, I simply imagined a patient sitting in front of me asking me what I was talking about. In the years I have been treating scleroderma patients, starting in 1981, I think I have gotten better about explaining what the disease is and what it does. I hope you agree.

I

INTRODUCTION
TO TERMS
AND
TYPES OF
SCLERODERMA

1
✳ ✳ ✳

WHAT IS
SCLERODERMA?

This book will tell you a lot about scleroderma. But there are two things it cannot tell you: the cause of scleroderma and the cure. These are the two most important things about any disease, and it is upsetting to the patient and frustrating for the physician that there are no answers to the most basic questions: "How did I get this?" and "How do I get rid of this?"

However, to say there is no *cure* for scleroderma is not to say that there is no *treatment*. There are many medications that can relieve the symptoms of scleroderma, and there are treatments that are promising in slowing or arresting the progression of the disease.

In this introductory chapter, I will present an overview of scleroderma and introduce some technical terms. I encourage you to get familiar with these terms because they will appear throughout the book and because you will encounter them over and over again in your doctor's office and in literature about this disease. Learning the language is the first step to understanding.

What is Scleroderma?

Scleroderma is an autoimmune connective tissue disease affecting blood vessels and collagen. One form (localized) tends to affect children, while the other (systemic) usually affects adults, although there are exceptions to this general rule. As you will learn, scleroderma is a disease characterized by exceptions.

Scleroderma can vary a great deal in terms of severity. For some individuals it is merely a nuisance; for others it is a life-threatening illness. My youngest patient was two years old when she developed the first "spot" that turned out to be morphea (a form of localized scleroderma). My oldest patient is now ninety-three. She was diagnosed fifty years ago with the systemic form of the disease. Between these two extremes of age are thousands of different stories and many different outcomes. No two stories are alike because the disease is expressed differently in different people and people respond in different ways. As with most things in life, there is no one "right" way to deal with this type of chronic disease. The purpose of this book is to give you information to demystify the disease, to give you a vocabulary to use when you discuss it with your family and with your doctor, and to help put you back in charge. This material is not meant to frighten you. If you are the type of person who sees herself or himself in all the worst scenarios, perhaps this book is not for you. If you are the type of person who is looking for answers, who feels that the way to get control is to learn as much as you can about your situation and to play an active part in your treatment, then please read on.

Classifying Scleroderma

In general, diseases are classified as (1) infectious, caused by organisms like bacteria or viruses, (2) genetic or inherited, caused by a defective gene and passed down from one generation to the next, (3) malignant or cancerous, (4) degenerative, referring to changes that come with aging, and (5) autoimmune, which means that the immune system is activated to attack the body's own tissue, rather than an outside organism. Scleroderma is classified as an autoimmune disease. This puts it in the same category as lupus (systemic lupus erythematosus, or SLE), rheumatoid arthritis, Sjogren's syndrome, multiple sclerosis (MS), and several others. The causes of all these diseases are unknown and none is curable, but all are treatable.

The term *scleroderma* means "thick skin." There are two kinds of scleroderma: the systemic form, which affects the internal organs or internal systems of the body as well as the skin, and the localized form, which affects a specific area of skin (see Table 1). There are also some conditions that are classified as sclerodermalike disorders because they share some features that are similar to scleroderma but have other features that are distinctly different.

As noted earlier, children with scleroderma usually get the localized form (further subdivided into linear scleroderma and morphea), while adults usually get the systemic form. There are exceptions to this rule, which will be dealt with in a later section.

Table 1 Types of Scleroderma

Scleroderma

A. Localized scleroderma (not involving internal body systems)
   1. Morphea
   2. Linear scleroderma
   3. Scleroderma en coup de sabre

B. Systemic scleroderma (involving internal systems)
   1. Limited scleroderma (sometimes called CREST)
   2. Diffuse scleroderma
   3. Scleroderma sine sclerosis

Sclerodermalike Conditions

A. Eosinophilic fasciitis (EF)

B. Sclerodema or scleromyxedema

C. Chronic graft versus host disease (GVHD)

D. Eosinophilic myalgic syndrome (EMS)

In systemic scleroderma, the activation of the immune system causes damage to two main body parts: the small blood vessels (called the vascular system) and the collagen-producing cells located throughout the body but concentrated in the skin In systemic scleroderma the small blood vessels tend to narrow, and sometimes the blood channel is totally closed. This is most marked in the fingers, which become overly sensitive to the cold as a result of the diminished blood supply. Small cuts on the hands are extremely slow to heal, and sometimes ulcers occur spontaneously.

Patients with systemic scleroderma are notoriously cold-sensitive (leading to thermostat wars in some households). It is this *vascular* part of the disease that is responsible for Raynaud's phenomenon (color changes of the fingers related to cold exposure), which happens in almost everyone (95 percent) with this form of the disease. It is also responsible for sudden rises in blood pressure that can lead to kidney damage (about 25 percent of patients). It is the *collagen* part of the disease that is responsible for the thick and tight skin, the lung problems, and the gastrointestinal features of the disease.

Localized scleroderma affects the collagen-producing cells of some areas of the skin and usually spares the internal organs and blood vessels.

Collagen

What is collagen? Collagen is a natural protein that is made by cells and deposited outside of the cell. It is what makes your skin firm, and it is the major component of connective tissue. Connective tissue is skin, tendons, joints, ligaments, and "capsules" around organs—it is what holds you together. When you get a cut, collagen is laid down to form the scar. If you have ever had a severe case of pneumonia that damaged lung tissue, the lung will heal with scar formation that can usually be seen on a chest X ray. This scar formation is an essential repair process of the body.

The problem in scleroderma is that cells start making collagen as if there were some injury that needs to be repaired, even though no such injury has occurred. And once started, the cells don't turn off. In systemic scleroderma this happens first in the skin, and then can occur in the lungs, the gastrointestinal tract, the muscles, and elsewhere in the body. This excess collagen gets in the way of normal functioning. The fingers don't bend well because of the collagen buildup in the skin; the lungs can't exchange oxygen for carbon dioxide effectively because there is a thick layer of collagen where a very thin membrane is supposed to be; the esophagus and bowel can't move effectively because there is scar tissue where muscle fibers are supposed to be.

Turning off these cells without damaging normal collagen formation is tricky. Under normal circumstances a small amount of new collagen is constantly being made while some old collagen is broken down. Laboratory researchers have successfully blocked all collagen production in laboratory animals, but the animals died. This is clearly not the answer. Slowing down collagen synthesis, enhancing collagen breakdown, or preventing the cells from becoming activated in the first place are approaches that are more promising. There is a great deal of research that is being done in these areas, but so far there has not been a great deal of success. If we knew the cause of scleroderma—that is, if we knew the trigger that started the whole process—then new treatments could be targeted to that early event. Since we don't know the root cause of this disease, doctors attempt to interrupt the process at various levels. These treatments can slow down the progression of the disease and can even arrest it in some patients.

Localized scleroderma is a much different condition. Excess collagen production is still the underlying problem, but it occurs as one or more patches of thick, tight skin anywhere on the body. This form is called morphea. In most cases, the patch or patches develop over a period of three to five years. After that, they tend to fade and the skin texture returns to normal, although there may be some pigment differences marking the old morphea areas as lighter or darker than the surrounding normal skin.

The other form of localized disease is linear scleroderma. This is an area of thickened and tight skin that develops in a "line" down one arm or leg or occasionally on the face. Usually only one such line develops. The tissue underneath this linear scar tends to waste away, and the scar can become very deep, extending down to the bone. When it appears on an arm or leg in a young child, it can interfere with growth of the limb. Sometimes there is an inflammation of the joints (swelling and soreness) under the scar as well.

The following chapters will discuss the different kinds of scleroderma in more detail.

2

✳ ✳ ✳

LOCALIZED
SCLERODERMA

*Limited, Localized, Diffuse, Generalized,
Systemic, and Not-So-Systemic:
What's In A Name?*

Scleroderma is divided into several different types, and the
terminology can be confusing:

Types of Scleroderma

A. Localized scleroderma (not involving internal body systems)
   1. Morphea
   2. Linear
   3. Scleroderma en coup de sabre
B. Systemic scleroderma (involving internal systems)
   1. Limited
   2. Diffuse
   3. Scleroderma sine sclerosis

It is easy to confuse localized and limited scleroderma—and sometimes even doctors get confused by these terms, since they certainly sound similar. But they refer to very different forms of the disease. I would much prefer that the entire terminology be changed for greater clarification, but I don't make the rules. This chapter will deal with localized scleroderma, and Chapters 3 and 4 will discuss the systemic form.

What Is Localized Scleroderma?

The word *localized* is used to indicate that this form of scleroderma is confined to a specific area of skin and does not affect internal organ systems. Localized scleroderma is more common in children than in adults. In my practice (which is mostly adults) the youngest child I have seen with morphea (a type of localized scleroderma) was three years old, although it can start in the first few months of life. My oldest morphea patient was eighty-six when it started and is now ninety. I mention this older patient to make two points: first, to give a sense that scleroderma can occur in all age groups, and second, as a reminder that when doctors employ terms such as "usually" or "for the most part," you have to keep in mind that there can be exceptions. Many of my patients get alarmed when they read medical information that seems to contradict their own experiences. They conclude that what has happened to them is not *supposed* to happen. To help put this into a nonmedical and perhaps more universal context, everyone understands the concept that it *usually* does not snow in Michigan after mid-April. However, sometimes it does. And with scleroderma, it can seem as if there are more cases with exceptions than those that follow the rules.

Morphea is a condition in which there are patches of thickened skin. These patches can range in size from half an inch to several inches. They can occur anywhere on the body. Sometimes there is a burning, itching, or stinging sensation that accompanies them, but frequently they are painless. The skin coloration is different from the surrounding normal skin, either lighter than normal (hypopigmented) or darker than normal (hyperpigmented). The initial spot is frequently dismissed by patients as a bruise from some minor injury that never quite healed. Only after it becomes noticeably thickened, or when another spot develops, is it brought to the attention of a physician. Sometimes there is only one spot, but frequently there are several, which develop gradually over a period of months or years.

The "typical" course of morphea in a child is that the spots develop over two to three years, then stabilize, then slowly resolve over the next few years. At their worst, the areas are thick and are noticeably different from surrounding skin. As they resolve, the skin patches return to normal texture, and by adulthood there is only a subtle difference in skin color that marks the place where the old morphea spots used to be.

This scenario is different in morphea that occurs in adults and in generalized morphea.

Scenario 1:
Adult Patients Who Had Childhood Morphea

Since I am trained in adult medicine, rather than pediatrics, I see children only occasionally. On occasion I consult with patients now in their twenties who come because they want a second opinion about their childhood morphea. The history usually is that their parents first noticed a spot when they were three or four years old, and it was subsequently diagnosed as morphea. By the time I see them, the spots are faded but still "findable." The issues at their visit are the following: (1) will the morphea reactivate (the answer is no), and (2) are they at risk to develop systemic scleroderma or another connective tissue disease like lupus (the answer is again no).

Scenario 2:
Morphea that Begins in Childhood

The milder cases of childhood morphea do not need to be treated, because the treatments have potentially serious side effects. If the morphea is spreading, with multiple spots, or if linear scleroderma is associated with it, then treatment is an option. Although clinical tests have not proven any medication to be uniformly effective in this condition, some patients seem to improve with the use of one or more types of treatment. Treatment can include the use of creams or ointments such as steroids (cortisone or cortisonelike medications), the injection of steroids into the morphea spots, and occasionally steroid pills. D-penicillamine, potaba, methotrexate, and others have been used. The approach is highly individualized.

Scenario 3:
Morphea that Begins in Adulthood

I have seen the onset of morphea in individuals from the late teens to age eighty-six. Most of the people I have seen have been bothered with a burning, itching, stinging sensation that signals a new lesion or the spread of an already existing one. Sometimes this feeling will begin before the skin appears abnormal, so they will know when a new spot or lesion is about to develop or when a preexisting lesion will enlarge. (The medical term *lesion* refers to any tissue abnormality, so there are skin lesions, lung lesions, brain lesions, benign lesions, cancerous lesions, and so on. It is a very general expression.)

About 30 percent of morphea patients will have a positive ANA (antinuclear antibody) blood test. An antibody is a protein that the immune system makes that usually attaches to bacteria or viruses and helps to eliminate them from the body. It is not known why some people make an antibody to part of their own cells (the nucleus), but this is characteristic of the autoimmune diseases, particularly scleroderma and lupus.

Morphea usually has no Raynaud's phenomenon (color changes of the fingers on cold exposure), a hallmark of systemic scleroderma. Additionally, there is no fingertip ulceration and no pulmonary or kidney problems, and only rarely are there any gastrointestinal problems. When GI problems do occur, they tend to be mild. For a comparison of localized and systemic scleroderma, see Table 2.

**Table 2   Distinctions Between
Localized and Systemic Scleroderma**

Localized Scleroderma	Systemic Scleroderma
No Raynaud's phenomenon	Raynaud's phenomenon in 95 percent
No fingertip ulcers	Digital ulcers in more than 50 percent
GI involvement rarely, except for generalized morphea	GI involvement in 85 percent
Positive ANA in 30 percent	Positive ANA in 80 percent

Scenario 4: Generalized Morphea

Generalized morphea is a condition in which most of the skin is involved, with patches of thickened and tight skin. These patches can be so extensive that they merge into one another. The patches usually start on the trunk or upper arms and legs and then spread down to the hands and feet. This is a pattern opposite to that seen in systemic scleroderma, which starts in the hands or feet and then spreads toward the central body.

Internal organ involvement is seen more frequently in generalized morphea than in simple morphea. It particularly affects the gastrointestinal tract, causing gastroesophageal reflux (heartburn symptoms), and less frequently causes lung and kidney problems. Since these complications are similar to the internal organ involvement in systemic scleroderma, I will refer readers to those sections. Diagnosis is made by skin biopsy and by the clinical appearance of the lesions.

Linear Scleroderma

The thickened skin of localized scleroderma can occur in patches (morphea) or along a line (linear pattern) on the head or down an arm or leg. Unlike morphea, linear scleroderma affects not just the skin and fatty tissue under the skin surface, but also underlying muscle and bone. This is particularly true in growing children.

If the line of sclerodermatous skin passes over a joint, for example, the knee or the ankle, it can limit the motion of the joint and lead to limb shortening. This is, of course, more of a problem in the leg and foot than in the arm, since leg length discrepancies and limited ankle motion can severely affect gait.

In almost all cases, linear scleroderma affects only one limb. Due to the potential of leg length discrepancies and gait problems, linear scleroderma of the lower extremity is usually treated. Treatment includes medications such as D-penicillamine (the name sounds like penicillin, but this drug is not an antibiotic), physical therapy to maintain range of motion and muscle strength, splinting of a joint to prevent *contracture*, and in some cases surgery. Contracture is a permanent bending of a joint so that it loses part of the range of motion. In scleroderma, contractures of the fingers result in bending in of the fingers toward the palm, or bending in of the elbow so the arm cannot be fully straightened out. As in morphea, the disease will go through an active phase, then stabilization, then a recovery phase in which the skin will return to a normal texture. However, growth does not "catch up" in the affected limb, and even though the overlying skin can lose its excessive thickness and return to a normal texture, the underlying fatty tissue may not return to normal, so the involved limb may always be smaller in circumference than the uninvolved limb. In many cases, the difference is fairly subtle.

When linear scleroderma involves the head, it may take the form of scleroderma en coup de sabre (*coup de sabre* means "cut of the saber"). Usually this starts as an indentation on the forehead or at the frontal hairline. Some hair may fall out in the area where the scalp is thickened. The line of thickened skin on one side of the face may spread to involve the entire face, down to the chin or neck. It does not continue down the body. There may be loss of the fatty tissue under the skin on the side of the face where the linear scleroderma is. This type of loss of tissue is called atrophy, and is named after two doctors who described the situation in the nineteenth century: Parry-Romberg syndrome or Romberg's hemifacial atrophy. Unfortunately, there is very little research into treatment for this condition.

Linear scleroderma can present different problems in adults, for whom growth is not an issue. The following case history, of a patient I'll call J.S., describes a fairly typical case.

J.S. first developed painful swelling in his left knee at the age of thirty-four. There had been no injury, and at first the concern was that his condition might be the beginning of rheumatoid arthritis. The knee pain improved with arthritis medicine, but then he developed a reddened area of skin over his left ankle. This gradually spread up his left leg. Over the course of a year, the thickened skin over his ankle prevented full range of motion, and the skin over his knee was so tight he couldn't fully bend the knee. He could straighten out the knee normally and was able to walk fairly well, but he had trouble running due to the restricted ankle motion.

Over the next three years, thickened skin developed on his thigh, with patches also on his abdomen (a combination of linear scleroderma and patches of morphea). With treatment, which included low-dose prednisone, D-penicillamine, and methotrexate, the signs of inflammation resolved and the skin gradually became thinner and more elastic. Range of motion at the ankle and the knee returned to normal, although the circumference of his left calf is an inch and a half smaller than the right calf. The skin of the left leg is somewhat darker than the right.

At its worst, which was about two years after the onset of the disease, J.S. developed muscle fatigue in the left leg and an aching sensation at the end of the day. Four years later, he is in the resolution phase of the disease and is able to play eighteen holes of golf. He feels that the left leg is still not as strong as the right, but he has no limitations on his activities either at work or during recreation. He has no internal organ involvement, although his ANA test is positive.

The arthritis in his knee never came back. It was present only at the onset of the scleroderma. The joint swelling is a little unusual in this case, but the overall course, from the onset of the first skin lesion (with signs of inflammation, including redness and discomfort), an initial phase of spreading skin involvement over about two years, and then gradual resolution with permanent loss of subcutaneous fatty tissue (the left leg is smaller than the right), is pretty typical. Did the medication do any good? When the dose was lowered, in an attempt to take him off it, the skin worsened. It then improved when the dose was increased again. Now that the skin is better, he has been able to stop two of the drugs and is on a low dose of the third with plans to discontinue it totally. I expect that he will be able to do this without a flare-up of his disease, since the scleroderma seems to have run its course.

Although not everyone is this lucky, this is a fairly typical scenario for linear scleroderma in adults.

3

✳ ✳ ✳

SYSTEMIC
SCLERODERMA—
DIFFUSE

The next two chapters will deal with the systemic forms of scleroderma, both diffuse and limited, as well as scleroderma sine sclerosis, in which there is internal organ involvement but no thickening of the skin.

The term *systemic* means that the scleroderma affects the internal organ systems. (Many textbooks use the terms *systemic sclerosis* and *systemic scleroderma* interchangeably; *sclerosis* means "hardening.") The terms *limited* and *diffuse* refer to the extent of skin involvement. Both forms are associated with internal organ damage, but the limited form tends to result in less severe organ problems than the diffuse form.

Limited scleroderma sometimes occurs as the CREST form. This is an acronym that stands for calcinosis, Raynaud's phenomenon, esophageal dysfunction, sclerodactyly, and telangiectasias—features that sometimes occur together. The following sections will deal with each of these features.

Primary Raynaud's Phenomenon

Raynaud's phenomenon (also known as Raynaud's disease or Raynaud's syndrome), is a condition in which the fingertips turn colors on cold exposure. Typically the fingertips first turn pale, then bluish or purplish, and then redder than usual. (In the United States, this is sometimes referred to humorously as "patriotic" color changes.) The color changes start to happen within seconds or minutes of cold exposure, and color returns to normal when the fingers are warm again. The fingers are usually numb for a period of time at the coldest point, and the patient sometimes feels a burning sensation as they warm up. Raynaud's phenomenon by itself (without scleroderma or lupus or other connective tissue disease) is very common, affecting about 5 percent of the adult American population. It is considered a "benign" condition, that is, one that is annoying but not disabling. I have even known some people with Raynaud's phenomenon in which the problem disappeared as mysteriously as it came. Many people who have it don't bother mentioning it to others, since they see themselves as unusually cold-sensitive rather than ill.

I remember being on vacation in Maine one summer with another family. We were swimming in a lake that was pretty chilly, and I remarked, rather cautiously, to my friend that her fingers appeared a little blue. I did not want to alarm her and I don't like making casual diagnoses, but it was a classic Raynaud's attack. She said she had Raynaud's, and not to worry about it, that her fingers always turned colors in the cold, and that her doctor had run some tests and said it was nothing to be alarmed about. I left it at that, because I thought her physician was correct; she did not have any of the hallmarks of scleroderma. Primary Raynaud's phenomenon does not cause sores or ulcers on the fingertips, is not associated with tight or thick skin, and really *is* something not to be alarmed about. If an individual has had Raynaud's phenomenon for two to five years and nothing else has developed, then it becomes extremely unlikely that an autoimmune or connective tissue disease will ever develop.

Secondary Raynaud's Phenomenon

Secondary Raynaud's phenomenon is a different story. A typical scenario in scleroderma is that Raynaud's phenomenon develops first and the person dismisses it, thinking it is just cold sensitivity. A year or two may go by without the person bringing it to the attention of a physician, especially if she or he feels otherwise healthy. Then, in a particularly cold period, a small fingertip sore may develop that just doesn't seem to heal. Everyone knows how tender a paper cut on a fingertip can be, and that it takes days for the cut to heal and the tenderness to go away. Well, these sores, although quite small— almost the size of a pinpoint—can take weeks to heal. This is the time when many people will go to their doctor. Frequently the skin over the fingers is already shiny and a little thick, but this process is so gradual that many people overlook it.

The diagnosis of Raynaud's phenomenon is usually made on the basis of the patient's description of the typical color changes and the fact that they occur suddenly after a short period of cold exposure. Some doctors will immerse the patient's hand in ice water in an effort to provoke an attack, but I think this is somewhat cruel and unnecessary. Frequently it is unsuccessful, too, since total body cooling is usually required for an attack to occur. Most often I see patients after they have been sitting in the waiting room for a while and have had a chance to warm up, but sometimes I'll see someone who has just come in from the cold. Then I'll bring in the medical students and the residents and tell them to look at the fingers and give me a diagnosis without talking to the patient (I only do this with patients I know). One of the great delights in being a medical school professor is that I get to stump the students—all in the name of medical education, of course.

Limited Scleroderma

Continuing the scenario outlined above, we see the onset of Raynaud's phenomenon occurring first, followed by the gradual development of puffy fingers and/or subtle changes in the skin of the fingers with some skin thickness (for example, rings get tight and may need to be resized). Often, this is brought to the attention of a doctor only when a small fingertip sore develops that is slow to heal. This process may unfold over two to five or more years. Characteristically, an individual will also notice heartburn on a frequent, usually daily, basis.

Heartburn is a symptom of stomach acid coming up into the esophagus, a process called gastroesophageal reflux (more about this in Chapter 7). It is felt as a burning sensation in the lower part of the chest, at the base of the breastbone (sternum). Most people have experienced heartburn after eating spicy food or a little too much food. Any woman who has been pregnant knows what heartburn feels like, as it is common in the last three months of pregnancy, especially on bending over or lying down, which causes the pregnant uterus to push on the stomach, forcing stomach acid to back up into the esophagus. Heartburn is such a common symptom that it is frequently overlooked by the patient and sometimes dismissed by a doctor or diagnosed as peptic ulcer disease. Many doctors will not think of scleroderma when a patient comes in complaining of frequent heartburn. Heartburn is common, scleroderma is rare.

Going back to our typical patient, we'll say she first noticed the color changes of Raynaud's phenomenon in 1990. Her fingers became puffy in 1993 and she began to have heartburn more frequently, causing her to start taking Tums on a regular basis. In 1995 she goes to her doctor because she has a sore on her finger that has been present for two months and just will not heal. Overall she feels pretty well, is going to work every day, and does not have the impression that she is particularly sick. All she wants is an antibiotic or some cream to help heal the sore. What she gets is a lot of questions, blood tests, and a referral to a specialist who will pursue a diagnosis of a connective tissue disease.

Diffuse Scleroderma

The situation is quite different for someone with diffuse scleroderma. The onset is faster and people usually do feel ill. Raynaud's phenomenon may not be the first symptom and, in fact, may never occur. It is hard to describe a single scenario that covers the onset of diffuse scleroderma, since there is a great deal of variation, so I will describe some general patterns of onset: (1) swollen hands and feet, (2) arthritis, (3) hypertension and renal failure, and (4) gradual development of thick skin over the limbs and trunk.

Swollen Hands and Feet

In this pattern, scleroderma starts with the swelling of the hands and feet. Many conditions other than scleroderma can cause swelling, or edema, particularly kidney problems and heart problems such as congestive heart failure. Additionally, some people will get foot and ankle swelling in hot weather, and many women notice some fluid retention resulting in puffy fingers just prior to their periods. Consequently, scleroderma is not the first thing a doctor will think of when a patient comes into the office complaining of swollen hands and feet. It can be a puzzling problem when all the tests are normal and no apparent cause is found. People are usually given diuretics, or "water pills," as a temporizing measure. It is a baffling situation if there are no other symptoms at this point of scleroderma, that is, if the skin texture of the hands and feet is normal (as is frequently the case in this stage), and there is no heartburn or other symptom of gastrointestinal or pulmonary (lung) involvement.

Frequently at this stage, people will have symptoms of carpal tunnel syndrome. Carpal tunnel syndrome is caused by pressure on the median nerve as it goes through a narrow "tunnel" at the wrist on the palm side. Symptoms include a tingling kind of numbness of the first three fingers that usually occurs at night and can awaken people from sleep. This numbness can also happen during the day and is relieved by shaking the hands. It is different from the numbness of Raynaud's phenomenon in that it is not triggered by cold exposure and it is not associated with color changes of the fingertips.

Carpal tunnel syndrome can develop from a variety of causes, and is frequently due to repetitive movements from working a machine or from typing. In severe cases surgery may be necessary. For those with carpal tunnel syndrome due to early scleroderma, the surgery may help the nighttime numbness, but it has no effect on the swelling. In fact, the swelling is caused by a "leakiness" of the small blood vessels in the hands, a result of damage to these vessels. The cause of the damage is unknown.

As time goes on, either Raynaud's phenomenon develops or the skin starts to get thick and tight, which suggests the diagnosis of scleroderma.

Arthritis

Some cases of scleroderma start out as swollen, painful joints of the hands, wrists, and other parts of the body. As you can imagine, this lands a person in a rheumatologist's office fairly quickly, and a diagnosis of rheumatoid arthritis is sometimes made, since at this stage there is no thick skin and no Raynaud's phenomenon. The picture can be somewhat puzzling, since the blood test for rheumatoid arthritis (the rheumatoid factor) is usually negative, but the ANA (antinuclear antibody) test is positive. The ANA usually, but not always, signals lupus or scleroderma. However, in rheumatology, the diagnosis is based more on the patient's symptoms than on what the blood test shows, and so a person with such symptoms is usually treated with arthritis medication.

It may be a few months or a few years before the characteristic skin features of scleroderma develop that permit an accurate diagnosis to be made.

Hypertension and Renal Failure

Sometimes scleroderma begins with the sudden onset of severe high blood pressure in a person with previously normal pressure and no prior diagnosis of scleroderma. The hypertension probably develops insidiously over a period of several days, and the first symptom is either a severe headache, signs of heart failure, kidney failure, or a stroke. The person is usually taken to the emergency room, where the high blood pressure is one surprise and the presence of kidney failure an even worse surprise. The key to treatment is to lower the blood pressure, which improves the kidney function. Sometimes the skin features of scleroderma develop *after* such an episode. In other cases, it is possible to determine that Raynaud's phenomenon had been present for a time or that some subtle changes in the skin of the fingers were present, but these signs were not considered to be important or significant.

Development of Thick Skin over the Limbs and Trunk

In some cases the thickening of the skin on the hands develops in a relatively short period, followed by extension of the skin thickness over the arms, with decreased motion of the fingers and wrists, in a matter of weeks. The changes are clear-cut and are brought to the attention of a physician fairly promptly. Reflux (heartburn) symptoms also occur, and there may be considerable joint pain and stiffness. The individual feels ill, with decreased energy, fatigue, and generalized muscle and joint aches and pain. This is the one form of presentation in which the diagnosis of scleroderma is made quickly. It is important to begin treatment promptly, to evaluate the degree and severity of internal organ involvement, and to monitor the patient's blood pressure and lung and heart function.

Treatment will depend on the degree and severity of inflammation in various organs.

Scleroderma Sine Sclerosis

Scleroderma sine sclerosis is a condition in which very typical scleroderma internal organ involvement occurs in the absence of skin thickness. Raynaud's phenomenon is usually present, which helps with the diagnosis, and the ANA is also positive. There is often a long delay (several years) between the onset of symptoms and the diagnosis of scleroderma because the main feature of the disease (thick, tight skin) is absent.

The treatment of this form of scleroderma depends on which organ system is involved, that is, the lungs, the gastrointestinal tract, the kidneys, and so on. People with this form of scleroderma should concentrate on reading the chapters that deal with their particular type of organ involvement.

4

* * *

SYSTEMIC
SCLERODERMA—
LIMITED

We left our patient with limited scleroderma in Chapter 3 at the point of being diagnosed. Let us pick up the story there and continue with the scenario. As you recall, she developed Raynaud's phenomenon (color changes of the fingers on cold exposure) in 1990, puffy fingers and chronic heartburn in 1993, and a fingertip sore in 1995. The sore prompted the visit to her doctor, who ordered lots of tests (what doctors do best) and referred her to a specialist. To make the story shorter, she is sent to a rheumatologist, without first seeing a hand specialist or a vascular specialist. By now the blood test results are known: the blood counts are normal, the kidney function tests are normal, the urine analysis is normal, the liver works just fine, the thyroid is normal, the cholesterol may be up a little, but in general the patient is fine on paper. The only test that is *not* normal is the ANA (antinuclear antibody) test, the screening test for autoimmune diseases such as lupus and scleroderma. The point of going to the rheumatologist is to find out which one it is and, therefore, what to do about it.

The rheumatologist makes the following assessment: middle-aged woman with Raynaud's phenomenon, sclerodactyly, fingertip ulcer, GERD (gastroesophageal reflux disease), and positive ANA. This certainly looks like scleroderma by the American College of Rheumatology criteria (see Appendix 1 for these criteria).

At this point there are three things that need to be done: (1) the extent of internal organ involvement needs to be determined (in lay language, more tests), (2) the diagnosis needs to be made more definitively to consider the possibility that this may be an overlap of scleroderma and other connective tissue diseases (in lay language, even more tests), and (3) the patient and family need to be told something. This last point is most important to the patient and most problematic to the physician. The patient wants definitive answers, whereas the doctor does not yet have all the information. Too much information will overwhelm the patient and may cause unnecessary anxiety. Too little information is unsatisfying and will create the impression that the doctor is uncaring.

My approach is to confirm that it is indeed scleroderma. I find that not having a diagnosis (and therefore fearing the worst) is more anxiety-producing than knowing the diagnosis. Then I tell the story of my ninety-three-year-old patient with limited scleroderma who was diagnosed at age fifty and is still living independently, although somewhat slowed down (due to her age, not to her scleroderma); she has outlived two of her doctors. I also inform people that this is rarely genetic, that is, they likely did not get it from their parents and cannot give it to their children (see Chapter 5). The rest—the specifics of treatment, the things to watch out for in the future—I put off until the results of the workup are known.

The workup usually involves the following: more precise blood tests to identify lupus and overlap conditions; pulmonary function tests; an electrocardiogram, or EKG (also known as an ECG); and a chest X ray if none has been taken in the past year. If there is difficulty in swallowing, as determined by the sensation that food sticks halfway down, or if there has been weight loss, then a barium swallow X ray may be done. If the patient describes heart palpitations, then a twenty-four-hour heart monitor may be used.

A few weeks later the patient comes back to my office for the results of the tests. The blood tests show that there is no evidence of lupus or overlap syndromes. The pulmonary function tests are either normal or show the results of smoking, not the pattern of lung involvement in scleroderma. The EKG does not show any abnormalities, and the discussion with the patient revolves around management of scleroderma symptoms.

There is no cure for scleroderma. Once you get it, you always have it. The disease can go into a phase of inactivity, in which nothing seems to be worsening, although problems with Raynaud's attacks and heartburn may persist. Some patients refer to this as a period of "remission." The point of treatment in the early phase, or at any stage of the disease, is to prevent complications from occurring and to relieve symptoms. All patients are different in that they have a different pattern of symptoms, so treatment regimens will vary from one patient to the next. For the patient described above, I will suggest a typical treatment program for this stage of her disease. Later chapters go into greater detail about different organ system involvement and the approach to treatment for each of these conditions.

Our patient here would benefit from the following: (1) treatment for the finger ulcer and advice about dealing with the cold to minimize the Raynaud's attacks, (2) treatment for the GERD (heartburn) to make her more comfortable and to prevent scar tissue buildup in the esophagus that can lead to trouble swallowing, and (3) information on what to look out for in the future.

Finger ulcers occur because the blood supply to the hands is decreased. This is also the cause of the Raynaud's attacks. Treatment is directed to opening up or dilating the blood vessels with a category of medication called calcium channel blockers. There are several of these on the market. Some of them are associated with side effects such as ankle swelling and light-headedness. As with most medication, the good effects have to be balanced by the side effects. Pentoxiphylline can be helpful in addition to the calcium channel blockers, but it needs to be taken three times a day. Low-dose aspirin (81 mg) is frequently used as well. There are some new medications being tested in experimental trials that may help, but as of this date they are not currently on the market.

Being careful to wear gloves and to dress warmly in cold weather is commonsense advice. Some of my patients keep little packets of chemical hand warmers (available at sporting goods stores) in their cars to keep their hands warm before the car heater warms up. There are some cars now that are equipped with heated steering wheels, an expensive but helpful gimmick. (Don't try to get the IRS to approve this as a deduction for necessary medical equipment; they do not have a sense of humor in this regard.)

It is *essential* that patients stop smoking. Nicotine and other substances in tobacco damage the small blood vessels and will only make the Raynaud's and the finger sores worse, not to mention doing damage to the lungs.

It is helpful to protect the sores by covering them with a loose Band-Aid-type cover. If an infection occurs, take an antibiotic for a week or so; it is not wise to be on antibiotics on a continuous basis, since this can result in bacteria that become resistant to medication. A dilute form of nitroglycerin ointment can be applied around the edges of the sores to improve blood flow. Warning signs that a skin ulcer is getting infected include the following: increased redness around the sore, increased swelling, pain and drainage, or red streaks up the arm.

For relief of the gastroesophageal reflux, there is a class of drugs called proton pump inhibitors that are extremely helpful. The reason to treat and prevent the reflux is not just to eliminate the symptom of heartburn, but also to decrease the possibility of breathing in some of the stomach acid when lying down at night. This can irritate the lungs and contribute to pulmonary fibrosis, or lung scarring. So, in addition to the medication, it is wise for the patient to follow antireflux precautions. These include not eating within two hours of bedtime, not lying down immediately after a meal, raising the head of the bed by about four inches, and eliminating foods that stimulate acid, such as chocolate and caffeine.

Pulmonary fibrosis, or buildup of scar tissue in the lungs, can occur in both limited and diffuse scleroderma. It can start several years after the onset of other symptoms even in people who have otherwise stable disease. Symptoms include a dry cough and gradual development of shortness of breath with activity. Treatment can slow down or reverse the fibrosis but is most effective if the scarring is caught early. Regular pulmonary function tests, done annually or biannually, can help to monitor this.

Kidney involvement, caused by a rapid and severe increase

in blood pressure, is uncommon in limited scleroderma, but it does occur in a small percentage of patients. To be on the safe side, individuals should have their blood pressure checked periodically. This is not as important for the patient with limited scleroderma as it is for someone with diffuse scleroderma.

After the initial diagnosis of scleroderma is made, patients need to be followed closely by their rheumatologist to monitor potential organ involvement and response to treatment. Individuals with stable limited scleroderma—that is, in whom the disease is not getting worse—should see their rheumatologist every four to six months. If new problems arise, they should be seen more frequently, of course.

II

EPIDEMIOLOGY: WHO GETS SCLERODERMA AND WHY?

5

✳ ✳ ✳

GENETIC FEATURES OF SCLERODERMA

Did You Get It from Your Parents?
Can You Give It to Your Kids?

Patients frequently ask me whether they can give this disease to their children. The short answer is no. While there may be a genetic susceptibility to scleroderma, for over 99 percent of patients no one else in the family has scleroderma. But let's take a closer look at who gets scleroderma and why.

Genes and Scleroderma

Diseases are classified as being genetic (inherited) or acquired. Inherited diseases are the result of an abnormal gene that gets passed down from one generation to the next. Acquired diseases are caused by exposure to some triggering factor that occurs at some point after birth. Some diseases occur through an interaction between an external trigger and an internal genetic predisposition.

Examples of diseases that are totally genetic (that is, passed down from one generation to the next) are sickle cell anemia, hemophilia (a bleeding disorder), and Huntington's disease (a nerve disorder). In these conditions, the only thing necessary to develop the disease is to inherit the gene. Usually these diseases become apparent in childhood, but sometimes (as in Huntington's disease) the first symptom does not occur until middle age. However, in all of these cases, there is a family history of other relatives being affected; sometimes several children in one family will be affected.

Other diseases are clearly acquired, like the flu. Several people in a family are affected at the same time. Since the time period is short between exposure and illness, it is clear that there is some "bug" or infectious agent that the family members are spreading among themselves.

Scleroderma is considered an acquired disease, that is, people are not born with it but develop or acquire it later in life. This means that they "catch it" somehow, from being exposed to something in the environment, perhaps a virus, a bacterium, a chemical, or an allergen (an allergy-causing agent).

Many diseases are caused by a combination of genes and environment. High blood pressure, or hypertension, is a good example, as is the tendency to have heart attacks. Hypertension and heart disease frequently run in families. But even if people have the gene, they do not have to get the disease if they are careful with their diet, exercise, medications to keep blood pressure and cholesterol levels normal, and other sorts of measures. Many of the diseases in modern life fall into this category.

Is there a gene for scleroderma? The answer, from what we know now, is that there probably is a susceptibility gene or several susceptibility genes, without which people could not get scleroderma. However, just having the gene is not sufficient; there must be some additional trigger to make the disease happen. There are examples from other diseases that could make this theory plausible. Rheumatic fever, for instance, is caused by the streptococcus bacteria that also causes strep throat. Strep throat is very common; almost every child develops it at some point. It is usually treated with penicillin or another antibiotic, which cures the problem. However, in some individuals, strep throat is complicated by the heart damage, high fevers, and joint swelling of rheumatic fever. The joint inflammation lasts about a month and then goes away, but the heart valve damage lasts forever and tends to worsen with age. Now that penicillin and other antibiotics are commonly used to treat strep throat, the incidence of rheumatic fever in the United States is much lower than it was fifty years ago. But even before the age of antibiotics, not everybody who got strep throat developed rheumatic fever. This was a puzzle for years, and it is only recently that researchers figured out that only those people who have a particular gene will get this complication.

What is the evidence that there is *any* role for genes in the development of scleroderma if most individuals have no family history of this disease? The evidence comes from an unlikely source: a group of Native Americans of the Choctaw tribe in Oklahoma who have a much higher than expected prevalence of scleroderma (almost eight times the prevalence in the rest of the country). These individuals have an unusual combination of immune regulation genes that non-Choctaws in Oklahoma do not have. One of the problems with labeling this gene complex as the "scleroderma gene" is that there are Choctaws who live in the southeastern U.S. who have this same unusual combination of immune-regulation genes but do not have this tendency to get scleroderma. The answer to this riddle is either that there is another gene (as yet unidentified) that the Oklahoma Choctaws have and the southeastern Choctaws do not have, or that there is something in the environment in Oklahoma that has triggered scleroderma in this group. The search is on for the gene, but this may give us only half of the story. Of course, half of the story is a lot better than none of the story, which is where we are now in our understanding of the cause of scleroderma.

An additional line of evidence for a genetic link comes from the few families in which more than one member is affected. Among the more than five hundred scleroderma patients I've seen, there are two families with scleroderma in two related individuals. One is a brother and a sister—he has diffuse disease and she has limited disease. The other family has two sisters affected. In both these situations, the diagnosis was made years apart, and long after these people had left home, so they had not shared the same environment for years. Could this have occurred by chance alone? This is pretty unlikely. Could this have happened *not* because of having a "scleroderma gene" but by being exposed to a particular virus or bacterium, which then stayed dormant in the body for years before emerging as scleroderma? We just don't know. We do know that viruses can remain in the body for decades and manifest years later as a disease that is very different from the original one caused by the virus. This is the case with chicken pox and shingles. Almost every child in this country gets chicken pox. Once infected, even though the pox "spots" go away in a few weeks, the virus stays in the nerve cells in an inactive state. Decades later it can reactivate and cause shingles, a very painful line of blisters that develop along a nerve pathway. The blisters will go away, but the pain can last for many months, and another attack of shingles can occur years later.

One way to distinguish between the role of genetics and the role of environmental factors is to study twins. If a disease is strictly genetic, then both members of a set of identical twins should have the disease. If the disease is strictly due to exposure (exposure here can mean a viral or bacterial infection, as well as exposure to a chemical or toxin) and if the exposure happened after the twins grew up and left the shared home environment, each twin should have only the same chance of getting the disease as the general population. (Actually, the best way to study this is to get twins who were separated at birth and therefore do not share any of the home environment, but this is extremely difficult.)

A study of twins, both identical and fraternal (nonidentical), was done by Dr. Timothy Wright and his colleagues at the University of Pittsburgh. They gathered blood samples from as many twins as possible, at least one of whom had scleroderma. What this group of researchers found is that the identical twins, who have identical genes, were no more likely to both have scleroderma than the nonidentical twins, who are no more closely related than any other brothers and sisters, but that this likelihood among all twins was higher than the likelihood in the general population. To put numbers on this, the likelihood of both twins in a twin pair having scleroderma was 6 percent, which is higher than what occurs in the general population, but nowhere near the 100 percent that would be expected if the disease was purely genetic. The conclusion from this, as from the pattern of the disease among Oklahoma Choctaws, is that there is some genetic component in scleroderma, but that there is something else in the outside world that a person must come in contact with in order to get the disease. I will discuss what little we know about this "something else" in the next chapter.

One final note about the twin study: This is an excellent example of collaboration among scleroderma researchers. I contributed a twin pair to this study, as did many other researchers around the country. We realize that solving the mystery of scleroderma will require this kind of cooperation and are hopeful that it will produce results soon.

6

✳ ✳ ✳

EPIDEMIOLOGY OF SCLERODERMA

Number of Patients, Occupational Links, and Environmental Connections

How many scleroderma patients are there? There has been some confusion and controversy over this number in the past. Previous studies of scleroderma were hindered by three factors: it is an uncommon condition, there was confusion over how to make the diagnosis (the criteria were established only in 1980), and there were few researchers interested in the disease.

Epidemiology is the study of the patterns of disease occurrence, that is, what the prevalence of disease is, how many new cases there are each year, and whether it is becoming more common. Epidemiologists study whether there are particular populations more likely to get a disease, for example, men versus women, one ethnic group more than another, or people in one country or geographic location more than those in another. By studying these patterns we can often identify risk factors that influence disease development and can help people prevent a disease by avoiding these risks.

For systemic scleroderma (including both the limited and the diffuse forms of the disease), the prevalence is approximately 240 cases per million American adults. This comes to about 80,000 patients in the United States. For localized scleroderma (including morphea and all its subtypes as well as linear scleroderma), the number is probably twice that for systemic disease, but accurate figures are not available. Overall, the number of *new* cases of systemic scleroderma is about 4,000 to 5,000 each year, and the number of *new* cases of localized scleroderma is about 6,000 each year. The number in the United States appears to be higher than that in Europe and Japan, although it is somewhat unclear if this difference is true or if it reflects differences in the methods of counting cases.

No definite answer can be given to the question of whether scleroderma is now more common than in the past, since really comprehensive studies have been done only in the past twenty years. However, in this relatively brief period, it does not seem that there are more new cases. However, the disease is becoming more widely known through the public relations work of scleroderma organizations and through the efforts of individual patients.

As for the third question, who gets this disease, I've already noted that women get scleroderma more frequently than men. Eighty percent of people with systemic sclerosis are women. This is also true for most forms of localized scleroderma, with the exception of linear scleroderma, which affects males and females equally. If more women get this disease, does this mean that female hormones play a role? Once again, the jury is still out. One study found that taking birth control pills did not affect the likelihood of getting scleroderma; taking female hormones to treat menopause did raise the likelihood of getting the disease, but only slightly. These two findings seem contradictory, and it is not clear what role, if any, female hormones play in disease development. It must be noted also that there is no evidence of any hormone imbalance in male patients, so right now the fact that scleroderma is more common in women remains an observation only, without a real explanation. Both rheumatoid arthritis and lupus are more common in women than in men, but hormones appear to have different effects in these two diseases. Pregnancy usually makes the symptoms of rheumatoid arthritis better, whereas pregnancy in lupus patients may make the disease worse. Pregnancy in scleroderma (see chapter 13) is considered a high-risk situation, although many patients do quite well.

There are particular ethnic groups that seem to have a higher incidence of scleroderma. African-Americans have a slightly higher risk of getting the disease, and this effect is most notable in younger age groups. Blacks tend to develop scleroderma at a younger age than whites and tend to have diffuse disease more frequently than whites. The reasons for this are not clear.

What about risk factors other than gender? Evidence for an association between scleroderma and chemicals or other materials in the environment, or particular occupations, is suggestive but not at all conclusive. Miners (coal miners in Pennsylvania and Germany, as well as gold miners in South Africa) have been reported to have an increased incidence of scleroderma. However, this does not explain the vast majority of cases, since very few women, and not too many men, are employed in mining. Out of my hundreds of patients, only one had an exposure related to mining, and this could have been coincidental.

Exposure to various chemical solvents also has been reported to be associated with scleroderma, but again, this does not account for the vast majority of cases.

It is natural for people to try to determine what caused their disease. It is very difficult psychologically and emotionally *not* to know what caused the disease. It is impossible to protect your family from getting it if you can't tell them what to avoid. The past twenty years of my professional life have been involved with solving this mystery. I hope that my next twenty years will not be spent similarly and that one day scleroderma will be relegated to textbooks on the history of medicine.

III

HOW SCLERODERMA AFFECTS THE BODY

7

✳ ✳ ✳

RAYNAUD'S PHENOMENON, SKIN INVOLVEMENT, AND FINGER SORES

This chapter relates to people with the systemic form of scleroderma, both those with limited disease and those with diffuse disease. It does not address people with localized scleroderma, which is morphea and linear scleroderma.

Raynaud's Phenomenon

Raynaud's phenomenon is a specific type of cold sensitivity that is characterized by color changes of the fingertips on cold exposure. There is some variation from one person to the next, but the typical attack starts with the fingertips getting very pale, then numb, and then turning a purple or blue color. This process starts within minutes of cold exposure and will last until the fingers get warm again. Sometimes the fingertips will turn red as they warm up; this can produce a throbbing or burning sensation.

As mentioned in Chapter 3, Raynaud's phenomenon is a common condition, affecting about 5 percent of the adult American population. Most of these people have primary Raynaud's phenomenon and will never develop scleroderma or other connective tissue disease. However, a small percentage of people will go on to develop scleroderma or lupus. In these people, the cold sensitivity is called secondary Raynaud's phenomenon. To make things even more complicated, some people with scleroderma do not have Raynaud's at all. However, most people with scleroderma do develop this cold sensitivity as the first sign or symptom that something unusual is happening.

The underlying process in a Raynaud's attack is a spasm of the small blood vessels in the fingers, causing the blue or purple color. The toes also are affected in many people, but the fingers are the most noticeable. These color changes are really an exaggeration of a normal response to cold exposure, since everyone will develop cold hands when they are exposed to cold for a long enough period of time. However, the normal cold response in the hands is a blotchy red and white pattern, and Raynaud's-type color changes are distinctively different.

How do you determine the difference between primary Raynaud's phenomenon and the secondary form? The distinction is made through a careful evaluation by your physician, who looks for features that would suggest either scleroderma or lupus. These include thickened skin on the fingers, difficulty swallowing, or frequent heartburn, in the case of scleroderma; or sun-sensitive skin rashes, joint problems, and other symptoms in the case of lupus. Additionally, a blood test (the

ANA, or antinuclear antibody test) is usually done. The diagnosis of either scleroderma or lupus is made when the patient has a combination of physical symptoms, usually in conjuction with a positive blood test. If the workup is negative for other signs and symptoms of these other diseases, and especially if the ANA is negative, then it is likely that the Raynaud's phenomenon is primary. However, sometimes it takes a while (two to five years) for the other features to develop, so most physicians will follow a patient for a few years before feeling comfortable assuring her or him that nothing else is likely to happen.

Sometimes I see people with Raynaud's phenomenon and a positive ANA, but nothing else, even after ten or more years of the typical color changes. I think these people also have primary Raynaud's phenomenon and should be reassured. The antinuclear antibody does not do anything bad by itself. It is only a marker for connective tissue disease. Also, the ANA does not distinguish between scleroderma, lupus, and mixed connective tissue disease. I wish I could explain this better, but I am hindered because not a lot is known about what makes this test positive to begin with. If it offers you any consolation, you now know almost as much about the ANA as your doctor.

Systemic Scleroderma and the Skin

The thickened skin of scleroderma is the most noticeable feature of the disease. As noted in earlier chapters, there can be only a limited degree of skin thickening, and this small amount can be missed by many doctors who are not familiar with the more subtle changes of scleroderma. The skin thickness can be limited to the fingers (called sclerodactyly) or can also involve the back of the hand, the forearm, the upper arm, the trunk, the legs, and the feet. It starts in the hands or feet and may or may not progress to involve other areas of the body. I have seen patients with all combinations of skin involvement. It is generally true that the skin thickening reaches its maximum extent within five years of the start of the thickening (not within five years of the onset of the Raynaud's changes).

As noted earlier, the word *scleroderma* means "thick skin." The thickness comes from an excess of scar tissue, which consists of collagen. Collagen is a normal component of skin, bones, cartilage, lungs, and just about every other organ in the body. It forms a sort of scaffold in which cells and organs reside. Under ordinary circumstances, collagen is a good thing.

In order to understand the role of collagen in scleroderma, and in order to understand the abnormality in this disease, we must discuss some basic cell biology. Formation of a scar is the body's normal response to damage done by trauma. Most of us have scars from old cuts or lacerations. Even internal organs can form scar tissue as part of the repair process. An example of this is lung scarring following a severe bout of pneumonia.

The normal sequence for the repair process after a laceration or cut that penetrates through the skin (that is, through both the epidermis and the dermis) involves several steps. The first response is bleeding and clot formation to "plug" the hole. Then cells in the dermis (called fibroblasts) become activated, actually move to the edge of the damaged tissue, and start making collagen. Under the microscope, collagen looks like a wavy rope or fiber. These fibers fill in the defect from the injury. Eventually the clot (scab) lifts off to reveal the scar underneath, and the structural integrity of the skin is restored. The activated fibroblasts either die off or return to a resting state, on guard for subsequent injuries.

How do the fibroblasts know that an injury has occurred, and how do they know where to go? This is an interesting question, because the answer to what triggers scleroderma is contained in the answer to it. While some substances, such as glucose and other nutrients, are always passing out of blood into tissue, blood is supposed to stay inside blood vessels, and fibroblasts are supposed to stay in tissue outside of blood vessels. When blood vessels are damaged, they release a large number of inflammatory substances, some of which activate fibroblasts and set in motion the repair mechanism of scar formation described above. (The white cells in the blood play a key role in releasing substances that activate fibroblasts; this is how the immune system is involved.)

In scleroderma, however, the fibroblasts become activated even though there is no apparent injury—no initial cut, no laceration. For some unknown reason and by some unknown mechanism, blood vessels spontaneously become "leaky," and skin fibroblasts start making too much collagen. This activation can occur in one or more small areas over several years (morphea). It can occur in a line down a limb (linear scleroderma), or it can occur beginning in the hands and progressing over the body, even including, to a varying extent, the internal organs (systemic scleroderma). No one knows what causes the blood vessel damage to begin with, what specific factors turn the fibroblasts on, and what will turn them off. No one knows why some people get a mild case, with skin thickening only on one hand, and others get skin thickness and tightness over the whole body. No one knows, either, why it is that some people get internal organ involvement (in the lungs, GI tract, or kidneys) without any external skin involvement. So I cannot answer your "why" questions, but I can answer some of your "how" questions. (I myself have been working on the "why" question since 1981, and I am confident that the answer will eventually be found.)

Skin problems in scleroderma can be grouped into six categories: (1) itching, or pruritus, (2) pigment changes, both darker skin and patchy areas of lighter skin, (3) skin ulcers, (4) skin thickness, resulting in joint contractures, (5) telangiectasias, or red spots, and (6) calcinosis (calcium deposits).

Itching

Itching, also known by the medical term *pruritis*, is a major problem for some people. It is caused by irritation in the skin from the underlying inflammatory process associated with scleroderma. It occurs without a rash, although some individuals will get a rash from scratching. The itching is worse at night (probably because the distractions of the day are fewer) and can be bad enough to interfere with sleep. For the most part, the itching occurs in the first two to five years of the disease and then subsides, although some people have problems with it for many years.

In terms of treatment, low-dose steroids (such as prednisone) can be helpful, but they have a lot of potential side effects, so this is usually considered a last resort. Antihistamines are somewhat helpful and have the added benefit of causing drowsiness. Creams and lotions may yield a temporary benefit but do not penetrate deep enough to provide prolonged relief.

Pigment Changes

Pigment (skin color) changes occur commonly in scleroderma. Some areas may have increased pigmentation (hyperpigmentation) and appear darkened, like a tan that doesn't fade, even though there has been no sun exposure. Other areas of skin may develop a patchy loss of skin pigment (hypopigmentation) in a "salt-and-pepper" fashion: On close inspection, the areas at the base of a hair follicle can be seen to have a spot of normal pigment while the surrounding areas have lost pigment. Sometimes this is mistaken for vitiligo, a skin disorder manifested by a smooth loss of pigment. Pigment changes can present a cosmetic problem. In some cases, prescription creams containing vitamin A (usually considered acne creams) can be helpful, but it can take months for them to have an effect, and these creams can be drying. For areas of the face and neck, makeup may be the only recourse. Over several years these changes can resolve and the skin tone returns to a more normal appearance.

Skin Ulcers

Skin ulcers are far more than a cosmetic problem. These usually occur on the fingers, either at the tips, due to poor circulation, or over the knuckles, where the skin is stretched tight. (Toe ulcers can also occur; both kinds are usually referred to in the medical literature as digital ulcers.) Sometimes a small cut or injury to the fingertip develops into a sore that will not heal because the blood supply is not good enough. Sores can occur at pressure points—for example, over the elbows—as well. Wherever these sores occur, they are painful and interfere with function. Treatment includes medication to improve the blood supply by dilating or widening the blood vessels (vasodilators), medication to help the red cells move through narrowed blood vessels (pentoxiphylline), cold avoidance, protection from the dozens of daily small traumas that can affect the fingers, keeping the area clean and dry, and constant vigilance against infection. Infections can occur in sores that are open for a long period of time, and these need to be treated with antibiotics. Because the underlying problem is usually the lack of blood supply, rather than an infection, the antibiotics alone will not cause the sore to heal. Once an ulcer develops, it typically takes weeks or months to heal.

The best way to treat these ulcers is to prevent them from happening in the first place by being cautious about cold exposure, which further reduces the blood supply to the extremities. Always wear gloves or mittens when cold exposure is likely, even in an unlikely place such as the grocery store. At first some patients feel self-conscious, but it does not matter what other people think. In the winter most of my patients keep little packets of chemical warmers in their cars to hold in their hands until the car heater gets going. It also helps to dress warmly, with an extra sweater or undershirt. There is no medicine that will completely eliminate the Raynaud's attacks, but there are several medications that can decrease the severity and frequency of these attacks. They belong to a class of drugs called calcium channel blockers. All medications have potential side effects, so you should discuss these with your doctor.

Primary Raynaud's phenomenon can be improved with biofeedback treatment. This is a technique in which a person learns to increase the blood supply to the fingers. Although biofeedback may be less helpful in the secondary Raynaud's attacks of scleroderma, it can be beneficial for some people. It takes a lot of practice and motivation. Biofeedback is usually taught by psychologists. Briefly, a small wire that measures temperature is taped to a finger. This is connected to a gauge that indicates to the patient if the finger temperature is going up or down. The person is then instructed to try lowering the temperature by imagining he or she is in a warm room, in a hot climate, and so on. The point is that with practice (usually at least ten sessions) most people can learn to raise their finger temperature. Practice is required until it becomes "automatic," so that the technique can be used on the spur of the moment. Biofeedback will not cure Raynaud's phenomenon, but in some individuals the technique can decrease the frequency and severity of attacks.

Sometimes finger ulcers occur in spite of careful precautions. In this case, it is important to be on medications to improve blood flow, to use antibiotics only if an infection has set in, and to be very careful to keep warm. In severe cases, surgery can be done to help free up the blood vessels at the base of the finger. This is called digital sympathectomy, and it removes the sympathetic nerves that are responsible for causing the blood vessels to go into spasm. This is very delicate surgery and there may be problems with healing of the surgical incision, so this procedure is usually reserved for the more extreme cases. In very rare cases, the tip of the finger may need to be surgically amputated in order to relieve pain.

Ulcers can also occur over the knuckles or over the elbows. This tends to happen due to a combination of poor blood supply and trauma—the frequent small injuries to fingers that happen every day, constant pressure from leaning on the elbows. The measures noted above (keeping warm, keeping the area clean, treating infections if and when they happen, using medication to improve blood circulation) are very important. Ulcers that occur on the lower legs or places other than those mentioned above are probably due to a different problem in the blood vessels, called vasculitis, which is treated with a different class of medication that reduces inflammation.

Skin Thickness Resulting in Joint Contractures

Skin thickness occurs in almost all patients with scleroderma and is the hallmark of this disease. In some individuals the extent and degree of skin thickness is fairly mild, affecting only the fingers. In those whose skin is moderately affected, there is thickness of the skin of the fingers, back of the hands, forearms, face, and lower legs. In others, thickness can involve the skin of the trunk (chest, abdomen, and back) as well as the skin of the face, arms, and legs.

In research studies of new drugs, the degree and extent of skin involvement is measured by a skin scoring system. The body is divided into areas (fingers, dorsum of the hands, forearms, upper arms, face, chest, abdomen, thighs, legs, and feet). Degree of skin involvement is determined by assigning a number (0 = normal, 1 = mild, 2 = moderate, or 3 = severe skin thickness). The numbers are then added together for a total skin score. The highest or worst score is 51. If the medicine under study is effective, then the skin score is expected to improve or get lower over time. Since some people will experience spontaneous improvement in skin score over time, a placebo group (those getting a "dummy" pill that does not contain the real medicine) is needed for comparison. Statistical analysis is done to determine if the people on the real medicine experienced a greater level of improvement than the people on the placebo pill.

Another way to objectively determine if the disease is improving or worsening is to measure the degree and extent of joint contractures. Since the fingers tend to curl inward (finger contractures) in scleroderma, the degree of hand extension is often used to gauge disease progression. This is done by having the patient extend her fingers (open the hand) as wide as possible and using a measuring tape to determine the distance from the tip of the thumb to the tip of the little finger. This is done over time and provides a fairly reliable and objective measure of hand function.

Sometimes the hair falls out in the areas of thickened skin over the arms and legs. This is due to increased collagen around the hair follicles in the dermis as well as to decreased blood supply to the follicles. One of the changes that heralds improvement in scleroderma is the regrowth of hair. Hair loss from the scalp can happen as well, but this is more characteristic of lupus and overlap syndromes (lupus and scleroderma or mixed connective tissue disease) than of scleroderma alone.

Telangiectasias

Telangiectasias are red spots caused by the dilatation (widening) of small blood vessels in the skin. In scleroderma these spots tend to occur on the hands and face. Usually they are simply a marker of scleroderma and by themselves cause no harm. Understandably, however, people don't like them, because they don't like having red spots on their face. These can be removed by laser treatment, but they tend to recur.

The only situation in which medical treatment is necessary (rather than cosmetic) is if the telangiectasias become

very large and bleed. In rare situations, these blood vessel mal-
formations can occur in the mouth, throat, or stomach and
cause significant bleeding problems. Laser therapy is the treatment of choice.

Calcinosis

Small calcium deposits can occur in the fingers, over the
elbows, over the knees, and in various other places. They start
out underneath the skin and feel firm. An X ray can confirm
that they are calcium deposits (they show up as white dots)
and nothing to worry about. They cause problems only if they
are in certain areas of the hands or fingers and get in the way
of hand function. Sometimes they break through the skin and
drain a white material. If open and draining, they can become
infected from the normal bacteria that live on the skin.

For the most part, I advise against surgical removal of
these calcium deposits because the incision site will be slow
to heal and because they tend to come back. At this point there
is no good way to prevent them from occurring. It does not
matter if your diet is high or low in calcium. The medications
for Raynaud's condition mentioned above, the calcium channel blockers, have been suggested as a treatment, but most of
my patients were already on these medications when the calcium deposits developed, so I don't think they are helpful.
Colchicine (a medicine usually used to treat gout) is sometimes helpful to treat the inflammation associated with these
deposits.

8
✳ ✳ ✳

SCLERODERMA
AND THE KIDNEYS

Kidney involvement occurs in about 20 percent of scleroderma patients. While the good news is that 80 percent
of patients will never get this complication, the bad news is
that it is difficult to predict which 20 percent will be affected.
Kidney problems occur most frequently in the first five years
after the diagnosis and tend to happen in those individuals
with diffuse skin involvement, that is, with skin thickness that
extends to the upper arms or the trunk. Although this is generally true, scleroderma kidney disease can affect others as
well. As I said before, throughout this book it will become
clear that there are many exceptions to the rule when it comes
to scleroderma patients.

Kidneys are damaged in scleroderma due to a sudden and
severe increase in blood pressure, referred to as malignant
phase hypertension. This is very unlike the usual kind of high
blood pressure, or hypertension, which tends to start gradually

and which results in organ damage such as strokes and heart attacks only after many years. In scleroderma, blood pressure can go from normal or even low normal levels to dangerously high levels in a matter of days, and kidney failure can occur in a matter of weeks. As with the "usual" type of hypertension, there are no symptoms in the early stages. After the first few days, the hypertension can cause persistent or recurrent headaches, nausea, and vomiting. If malignant phase hypertension continues uncontrolled, kidney function can be lost and can progress to total kidney failure. Once this happens, dialysis is necessary.

The way to prevent kidney damage is to detect and treat the scleroderma-related hypertension as soon as possible. Patients who are considered to be in the high-risk category should invest in a home blood pressure apparatus and measure their pressure on a regular basis. Twice a week is considered often enough. If the pressure starts to go up, then it should be taken on a daily basis. If the blood pressure stays elevated for three days in a row, then your doctor should be contacted. How high is too high will depend to some extent on what a person's blood pressure normally runs. In this case, the lower number, or diastolic measurement, is considered the more important indicator of elevated blood pressure.

If malignant phase hypertension occurs and is caught early, the blood pressure can be brought under control with medication, usually ACE inhibitors (angiotensin-converting enzyme inhibitors). Other types of blood pressure medications tend not to work as well as the ACE inhibitors and will not prevent the onset of this problem. If the pressure does start to go up, it is very important to get it down to normal levels as quickly as possible. This will require frequent blood tests to monitor kidney function, and adjustment of medication doses as required. Sometimes this can be done as an outpatient, but occasionally, at least with the first episode of hypertension, patients will need to be hospitalized.

Once kidney function is lost, dialysis becomes necessary to maintain life. Dialysis is a process in which blood is removed from the body and passed through a special membrane that removes the waste products from the body, which the kidneys normally remove. The filtered blood is then put back into the patient. This process takes about four hours and is usually done three times a week. One of the difficulties with dialysis is that the dialysis machine does not do as good a job as normal kidneys, and people don't feel as well as normal. In some cases of scleroderma renal failure, some kidney function can be regained and the person can go off dialysis if the blood pressure is kept under control.

However, if kidney failure persists and long-term dialysis is needed, a kidney transplant can be done. There is the concern that hypertension will come back and ruin the transplanted kidney. However, the immunosuppressive medication used to prevent rejection of the kidney transplant will help to keep the scleroderma under control. And, of course, the blood pressure must be carefully monitored and controlled.

Clearly not every headache and not every episode of nausea or vomiting represents an episode of uncontrolled high blood pressure. This is why it is important to have a blood pressure cuff at home and know how to take your own pressure. For individuals who have limited scleroderma (skin tightness limited to areas below the elbows and below the knees), it is not necessary to take frequent blood pressures.

Once a person has had problems with scleroderma-related hypertension and gotten it under control with medication, it may be possible to decrease the dosage and in some cases go off the medication entirely. In this case, the pressure should be monitored frequently (again, twice a week). These individuals are at risk for repeated episodes of hypertension. If caught early and treated immediately, the pressure usually returns to normal and there is no damage to the kidneys.

The difficulty, as you probably have already figured out, is in promptly identifying and treating the *first* episode of malignant hypertension. As noted above, since this problem occurs in only a small number of patients who are at risk for several years, what is the best advice to give someone in order to strike a balance between reasonable safety and unnecessary worry? I recommend that you speak to your own doctor to find out if you are at high risk of developing this form of high blood pressure. If the answer is yes, then you should learn how to take your own pressure and find out at what pressure level you should be concerned and notify your doctor. For the most part, it will be reassuring to know that your pressure is normal.

Blood pressure normally fluctuates quite a bit on a daily basis and from day to day. For most people, the pressure is lowest in the morning and rises with activity during the day. I usually recommend that my patients take their blood pressure around the same time every day. It really does not matter what that time is, and I give them a range of normal pressures, approximately 100–150 (systolic) over 60–90 (diastolic). A single reading of 160/92 should not cause alarm, but should indicate that the pressure should be taken on a daily basis for the next few days. If the pressure stays at this level for three days in a row, especially in someone whose blood pressure is normally in the 100/60 range, then treatment should be started and the patient watched very carefully. On the other hand, if someone's blood pressure is usually 150/88, then the allowable levels will be different.

What about those people who have scleroderma and, coincidentally, have the usual kind of high blood pressure? Scleroderma is rare, but high blood pressure is very common in the United States, and the two conditions will overlap in some people just by chance. Actually, it is easy to tell the difference. Scleroderma-related hypertension occurs abruptly, and once elevated, the blood pressure continues to climb and can go to very dangerous levels that can result in a heart attack or a stroke. Also, blood tests that measure kidney function are abnormal. Usual hypertension, on the other hand, tends to remain at about the same level day after day, and kidney function tests are normal for years.

On rare occasions, scleroderma will start with an episode of malignant phase hypertension, and the other features of scleroderma (Raynaud's phenomenon, skin thickness, GI problems) happen afterward. In such cases, there is no reasonable way to detect the problem early.

9

✳ ✳ ✳

SCLERODERMA AND THE GASTROINTESTINAL TRACT

This information applies to people with systemic scleroderma, either limited or diffuse, and those with scleroderma sine sclerosis. It does not apply, or only rarely applies, to people with localized scleroderma (the morphea or linear type).

Background: How the GI Tract Works

Almost everyone with systemic scleroderma (about 85 percent of cases) has some degree of GI (gastrointestinal) tract involvement, from mild to severe. The GI tract includes the esophagus, the stomach, the small bowel or intestine, the large bowel or colon, and the rectum (see Figure 1 on page 68). It is made up of a special kind of muscle called smooth muscle, which is different from the striated (skeletal) muscles in the arms and legs. The main pathological process that happens in the GI tract in scleroderma is that the normal smooth muscle tissue is replaced by fibrotic scar tissue, a result of the fibroblasts' excessive production of collagen.

Smooth muscle is not under conscious control like skeletal muscle, but is automatically controlled through a system of nerves called the autonomic nervous system. The purpose of the GI tract is to propel food and fluid in one direction from the mouth to the rectum. It begins with the swallowing mechanism in the upper throat, which forms the transition between controlled motion in the mouth, the semicontrolled motion of initiating swallowing, and the automatic motion of taking the swallowed material into the stomach. We all have had the sensation of chewing something and starting to swallow and then being able to stop swallowing and bring the food back up to the front of the mouth by clearing the throat or coughing. That is, we blow air up from the lungs to propel the food out of the back of the throat. Once the food is beyond this point, however, it cannot be brought back up easily. Once food is swallowed, the reflexes from the autonomic nervous system coordinate the contraction of the muscles so that food is propelled efficiently through the esophagus to the stomach. There is a special structure at the gastroesophageal (GE) junction (the place where the esophagus joins the stomach) called the lower esophageal sphincter. It prevents the stomach contents from going backward up the esophagus. This does not seem like much of a feat, since people usually eat sitting up and gravity alone would direct food into the stomach. However, consider the situation of someone lying down and eating. If the muscles work normally, what is swallowed still gets to the stomach. As a matter of fact, if this system is working properly, people can stand on their heads and not have stomach acid travel up (or in this case down) the esophagus into the mouth.

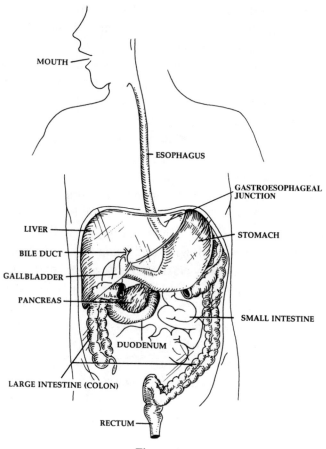

MOUTH

ESOPHAGUS

GASTROESOPHAGEAL JUNCTION

LIVER

STOMACH

BILE DUCT

GALLBLADDER

PANCREAS

SMALL INTESTINE

DUODENUM

LARGE INTESTINE (COLON)

RECTUM

Figure 1

The normally working esophagus, therefore, propels food and fluid down the esophagus, through the GE junction (one way only), and into the stomach, where it mixes with stomach acid, which starts to break down the food into smaller segments that can be absorbed. The stomach contents are emptied into the first part of the small bowel, called the duodenum, and pass by the common bile duct, which adds bile salts to break down fats and also pancreatic enzymes to break down protein and carbohydrates. All of this continues on down the length of the small bowel, where the lining cells that form the mucous membrane start to absorb all the good stuff (nutrients) and let pass all the indigestible stuff (roughage). The roughage gets dumped into the large bowel or colon, which is the first place in this process that involves bacteria. The gut, from the level of the stomach through the small intestine, is usually sterile, due to the action of the acid and the enzymes in the stomach juice and bile. This is pretty strong stuff and is capable of killing most bacteria and many viruses.

The large bowel does two things: It absorbs water, and it utilizes normally occurring bowel bacteria to break down the bile salts, which are reabsorbed and recycled. The rectum holds the fecal material (feces or stool, in medical terms) until it is released by the muscles of the anus, which are back under conscious control.

Now let us consider some pathological or disease conditions that change this smoothly functioning mechanism. First let us look at what happens with a common viral infection like the flu. As I mentioned above, many but not all viruses are killed by stomach acid and bile. Some viruses are not killed but pass through the GI tract without causing trouble. But there are particular viruses that are specially adapted to latch on to the cells of the mucosal lining (the lining of the GI tract) and infect them, leading to viral gastroenteritis, sometimes called stomach flu. The body, in an attempt to get rid of the virus, speeds up the motion of the bowel (called peristalsis). This results in diarrhea, which gets rid of the material in the intestines. The body may even reverse the normal direction in the upper tract, vomiting material from the stomach and even, sometimes, from the duodenum. You may feel miserable, but the autonomic nervous system is doing what it is supposed to do under the circumstances, which is to get rid of the virus as soon as possible.

Another common problem in the general population is constipation. The most common cause of constipation in our society is lack of adequate fiber in the diet and not drinking enough water. Lack of exercise contributes as well. But in scleroderma, alternating diarrhea and constipation can occur from a different combination of circumstances, which I'll discuss shortly.

Reflux

Gastroesophageal reflux disease (GERD) is the most common GI problem associated with scleroderma. The primary symptom of reflux is heartburn. This is a painful, burning sensation felt near the bottom of the breastbone (the sternum). Since the stomach tends to lie on the left side of the upper abdomen, the burning frequently seems as though it is coming from the left side of the chest and can be mistaken for chest pain coming from the heart, hence the term *heartburn*. The burning is actually caused by stomach acid flowing backward (*reflux* means "backward flow") into the esophagus. Whereas the lining cells of the stomach are especially suited to withstand stomach acid, the lining cells of the esophagus are not and can be damaged by persistent or recurring acid reflux.

How do you tell if a burning sensation near the breastbone is due to scleroderma or to normal heartburn, a common experience in the general population? There are some situations in which heartburn is so common it is considered normal. For example, during pregnancy, smooth muscle tissue relaxes, making the GE junction less tight, and the pregnant uterus also pushes against the stomach. Consequently, when a pregnant women bends over or lies down, she can experience heartburn. Additionally, the lower esophageal sphincter at the GE junction tends to weaken with age, so heartburn becomes more common as people get older. Being overweight with more fat in the midsection will also contribute to reflux. A hiatal hernia, in which part of the stomach extends into the chest through the diaphragm, will cause heartburn. Many people experience heartburn if they eat particularly spicy foods because the spices stimulate stomach acid production.

However, the reflux associated with scleroderma is different from the above situations in that it occurs on a daily basis, usually several times a day, regardless of the type of food eaten. This situation is a clear-cut change for the individual. Reflux or GERD associated with scleroderma is caused by the weakening of the muscles at the lower end of the esophagus, which normally prevent stomach acid from coming back up.

Dysphagia

With continued reflux over time, scar tissue can build up and cause the swallowing passage to narrow. This narrowed area is called a stricture. Patients complain that they eat a small amount and the first few bites may be okay, but then something seems to get "caught." Sometimes they can force the food down by drinking water. Other times the only way they can relieve this feeling is to make themselves throw up. Many people will consciously or unconsciously change their diet so they don't eat large bites of meat or even large chunks of bread, or they always drink a lot of liquid as they eat and chew food thoroughly. Some people will change to an almost totally liquid diet to avoid this problem. I had one patient whose weight dropped to ninety pounds due to an esophageal stricture that caused her to switch to a liquid diet. After an esophageal dilatation (opening) with an instrument called an endoscope, she was able to eat normally and gained forty pounds, returning to her usual weight.

Occasionally trouble swallowing (dysphagia) occurs even without formation of a stricture. Food seems to "hang up" in the esophagus. This occurs because there is ineffective peristalsis or muscle power to propel the food into the stomach. The muscles of the esophagus are replaced by scar tissue. Sitting upright to eat, eating slowly, chewing food thoroughly, and drinking fluid with the food are all good strategies to help with this. The way to determine if this is happening, or if there is an esophageal stricture, is to do a special X ray called a cine esophagram. This is a procedure that uses a motion-picture camera to record the contractions of the esophageal smooth muscle as the patient swallows a drink containing barium. There is a distinctive pattern in the scleroderma-affected esophagus that differentiates it from a hiatal hernia and that helps to make the diagnosis. A stricture is readily seen with this X ray as well. If the diagnosis of scleroderma is firm and the only reason to do the test is to see if a stricture is present, then a simple barium swallow will be adequate without the motion-picture part.

In addition to strictures, ulcers can occur in the esophagus from acid damage. These can make swallowing painful. Reflux of stomach acid can occur not just when eating, but at any time, especially on lying down. Small amounts of stomach acid can come back up the throat when people are sleeping and can be breathed into the larynx, causing damage to the vocal cords and a hoarse voice and/or sore throat in the morning. Stomach acid can sometimes be breathed into the lungs, contributing to lung irritation and lung fibrosis. Clearly there are many reasons to treat this condition.

Esophageal spasm (a sudden contraction or cramp in the esophagus) can occur due to a combination of many of these problems. This is a sudden and very painful condition resulting in severe chest pain and pressure. Most of my patients who have experienced this have gone to the emergency room, afraid that they were having a heart attack. Only after the doctors conclude from EKGs and blood tests that the heart is okay can they determine that the pain must have been coming from another source such as the esophagus.

Barrette's esophagus is a precancerous condition resulting from chronic inflammation of the lower part of the esophagus. As mentioned above, the cells that line the esophagus are not adapted to a highly acidic environment, as are the stomach lining cells. In some cases, the body responds to this chronic acid irritation by changing the cell type of the esophagus. Although these cellular changes are not a true cancer in the early stages, their presence means that there is an increased probability that cancer will develop. In this situation, annual endoscopy and biopsy are suggested. This involves examination of the esophagus and taking a sample of cells. Like most cancers, if detected early, treatment can lead to a cure.

Painful swallowing can be caused by an esophageal stricture or esophageal spasm, but for people on antibiotics, the possibility of a yeast infection of the esophagus (candida esophagitis) should be considered. The diagnosis is made by endoscopy. If present, the yeast infection can be cleared up with a special antifungal drug.

Occasionally scleroderma patients will have an infection in the stomach with a bacterium (*Helicobacter pylori*) that is the most common cause of ulcers in the general population. There is now a blood test to check for this infection. The point of getting the test is that if the infection is present, symptoms will improve with antibiotic treatment, though this will not eliminate the scleroderma-related scar tissue in the esophagus, stomach, or bowel.

Treatments for Reflux

There are now excellent medications on the market to treat reflux. These are called proton pump inhibitors, which are frequently superior to the usual ulcer medications. Additionally, medicine that stimulates the action of smooth muscle (called prokinetic agents) can be used in conjunction with the proton pump inhibitors to treat reflux. Remember, the goal is not just to prevent the discomfort of heartburn, but also to avoid the development of esophageal ulcers, strictures, vocal cord irritation, and possible lung fibrosis.

For the above reasons, even if they are on medication, patients should observe the following reflux precautions:
1. Don't eat within two hours of bedtime
2. Eat sitting up, eat slowly, and chew food carefully
3. Drink sips of water between bites and make sure each mouthful is fully swallowed before taking the next bite
4. Elevate the head of the bed at least four inches, using bricks or old phone books, for example. Do not simply elevate your head with a couple of pillows; you will slide off at night, and the angle of your head and body may make the reflux worse.

The treatment for esophageal spasm is, surprisingly, the same as the treatment for angina (angina is true heart pain, caused by a decrease in blood supply to the heart muscle), and that is nitroglycerin tablets under the tongue. However, I recommend this only after the patient has had a thorough workup for heart disease and it is clear that the chest pain is not coming from the heart.

Although most people with scleroderma (about 85 percent) will have esophageal problems to some degree, not all will have severe problems. Many patients will have only mild reflux symptoms even after many years of scleroderma. It is impossible to accurately predict who will have bad problems and who will have only mild involvement. One of my goals in writing this book is to include all, or virtually all, of the possible problems that could develop, so that every scleroderma patient could find herself or himself in these pages. In almost twenty years of taking care of hundreds of patients, I have never yet seen one patient with *all* these complications.

Problems of the Stomach and Small Bowel

The stomach can be involved in scleroderma in several ways: (1) the stomach is slow to empty, leading to a sense of feeling full after eating only a small amount, frequently accompanied by nausea, (2) erosions or ulcer formation occur as a result of acid buildup and sometimes as a consequence of medications, and (3) telangiectasias, or dilated blood vessels, that can bleed are present in the stomach. This last condition has been dubbed "watermelon stomach" due to the striped appearance of the dilated blood vessels as seen on endoscopy. The treatment for the first two conditions is the use of proton pump inhibitors or ulcer medicines coupled with the prokinetic agents mentioned above. The treatment for the third condition may include the use of female hormones, which have the unexpected effect of shrinking these blood vessels. In some cases the blood vessels can be cauterized (using an electric current to cause them to close off) through the endoscope. In severe cases surgical removal of part of the stomach is required.

As the muscle of the small bowel becomes replaced by scar tissue, the bowel tends to slow down. The first symptom may be a sense of bloating after eating, a sign that food is slow to move along the GI tract. People may complain of increased gassiness. There may be cramping, which is caused by an unusually hard contraction of bowel muscle in an attempt to force material through. Pain in the bowel is usually caused by distention or expansion of one segment. Swallowed air or gas from bacterial digestion can get caught behind food material that gets "stuck" due to the slow transit. As this gas expands, it triggers the pain receptors.

Some people with constipation do well on a high-fiber diet, but others think that this worsens their gassiness. Foods such as beans, which are high gas producers, should be avoided. Exercise—for example, walking after meals—helps promote motion in the bowel. A stool softener containing sodium dodecyl sulfate can be helpful. (There are several brand names; talk to your pharmacist.) For the most part, laxatives should be avoided. These may help the problem in the short run but can make constipation worse in the long run. If you do use laxatives, consult your doctor and have a plan to minimize their use.

The preceding sections explain why people with scleroderma get constipated. But why does diarrhea happen?

As mentioned above in the section on how the normal GI tract works, the small bowel is normally free from bacteria. When the motion of the bowel is slowed, however, bacteria from the large bowel can spread backward into the small bowel, creating a situation called bacterial overgrowth. These bacteria then break down the bile acids that are needed for fat digestion; the result is that fats cannot be absorbed, causing diarrhea and weight loss. The process is called malabsorption. The diarrhea can go on for weeks or months and cause considerable loss of weight. One of my patients went from 240 pounds to 140 pounds over a fifteen-month period. This type of weight loss can result in vitamin deficiency, which in turn leads to many other problems. The treatment for this kind of diarrhea is much different from that for the usual type of diarrhea, which comes with the flu or food poisoning. Most of the ordinary types of diarrhea will go away on their own after a few days. However, the diarrhea from bacterial overgrowth should be treated with a course of antibiotics; consult your doctor. For this problem it's best to take antibiotics for a short period of time, ten to fourteen days, followed by a period of a few weeks off medication, followed by another two weeks or so of treatment. Sometimes the diarrhea can be controlled after a few rounds of this type of therapy, and people can go for months or years without another treatment cycle. Occasionally people need to be on some form of antibiotics almost continuously. Another strategy involves finding out whether particular foods make the problem worse. Some people find that dairy foods will exacerbate the diarrhea. In those cases, avoidance of milk, ice cream, and cheese is a good idea. Since these foods are an excellent source of calcium, I do not recommend their avoidance to everyone. I suggest a trial-and-error system to see what works for you.

This is another situation in which the prokinetic agents are used. These medications can be very helpful in improving the motion of the bowel muscle that is left, but once the fibrosis reaches a severe level (which, fortunately, happens only in rare cases), there is not enough muscle left to stimulate. In addition to pills, there is an injectable medication called somatostatin that can be helpful in very severe cases.

If the bowel problem doesn't respond to these approaches, there are two options. The first is tube feeding with an elemental diet, which is a solution of ready-to-absorb protein, fats, and carbohydrates with added vitamins and minerals. It tastes truly horrible and is meant to be taken through a tube directly into the stomach or small bowel. However, in individuals whose small bowel is not capable of handling even this fluid, the only alternative is intravenous feeding using an indwelling IV line, usually inserted into the large vein under the collarbone. The special IV lines are meant to stay for months at a time, and the IV solution can be hooked up periodically throughout the day. Difficulties arise in that all the connections must be kept sterile, and the IV tube can get clotted off, requiring a replacement. Over the past twenty years I have had only a handful of patients (out of almost six hundred) who have required intravenous feedings because their GI tract simply would not move food along.

The Large Bowel

Involvement of the large bowel usually manifests as constipation. On testing with a barium enema, large outpouchings called diverticuli can be seen. These seldom if ever cause diverticulitis, which is an inflammation of a smaller type of outpouching that tends to occur in some people as they get older. The treatment for this type of constipation is the same as for constipation of the usual variety, that is, stool softeners on a regular basis, a diet with adequate fiber (avoiding high-fiber foods that are high gas producers), exercise such as a walking program, and the cautious and only occasional use of laxatives.

Another cause of constipation is hypothyroidism, or an underactive thyroid. This is more common in scleroderma patients than in the general population, so a blood test for thyroid function should be done to consider this possibility. If the thyroid is not functioning properly, supplemental thyroid hormone should be taken. This is available in pill form.

Anemia from Bleeding in the GI Tract

Anemia, or low hemoglobin in the blood, can occur in scleroderma patients as a direct result of the scleroderma itself, in which case it is called anemia of chronic disease, or as a result of blood loss through the GI tract. This is most frequently caused by bleeding from esophagitis or esophageal ulcers, from stomach ulcers, or from the dilated blood vessels in "watermelon stomach." The best approach is to identify the source of the bleeding with one of the tests mentioned at the end of this chapter and direct treatment toward that particular problem. Sometimes transfusions are necessary if the anemia becomes severe. Iron supplements can help if the anemia is due to blood loss and not to the anemia of chronic disease. However, iron tends to be hard on the digestive tract and can cause nausea, vomiting, abdominal cramping, and diarrhea on its own.

Coordinating Your Care

So who is your doctor under these circumstances—your rheumatologist or your gastroenterologist? Since scleroderma can affect many organs and since no one doctor can do all the procedures you may require, you will end up with a series of doctors. Sometimes one doctor will tell you one thing and another will tell you the opposite. What you need is a "quarterback," one person to do the coordinating, to know all the medications you are on, and to make sure they are not in conflict. This is usually the rheumatologist, but you need to decide along with your doctor who this will be. Managed care plans can sometimes make it difficult to get referrals, but you have to get in the driver's seat. You (yes, you) have to make sure that reports are sent from one doctor to the next. It may be necessary for you to ask for a copy for your own personal records and then make sure that copies are distributed to all your doctors. It is okay to request this, and you don't have to be able to understand what the reports say.

✳   ✳   ✳

At right is a summary of the tests that are available and frequently used in scleroderma. I certainly do not use all these tests in all patients with GI problems. Sometimes the situation is so clear that I feel I don't need to do any testing. As a general rule of thumb, I order tests when the clinical situation is not clear-cut or when another disease or condition can be present that would require a different therapeutic approach.

Summary of GI Tests:

Barium swallow: an X ray test that can determine if a stricture is present in the esophagus or if there is a hiatal hernia; this requires swallowing a liquid with barium dissolved in it (barium shows up white on an X ray)

Cine esophagram: an X ray test similar to the barium swallow that takes an X ray movie of the motion of the esophagus; this can determine if there is decreased motion of the esophageal muscles of the type seen in scleroderma

Upper GI series: a barium swallow that follows the barium through the stomach into the small bowel; it can also pick up some stomach ulcers or tumors

Transit study: the measurement of the time it takes for material to go from the stomach through the bowel

Hydrogen breath study: a test to determine how much of a sample meal is absorbed; this can determine if there are bacteria in the small bowel, so this is a test for malabsorption

Upper endoscopy: a test in which a tube (endoscope) is passed through the mouth into the esophagus and stomach so that the doctor can see the lining of the esophagus and stomach, and inflammation, ulcers, enlarged blood vessels, bleeding sites, and tumors can be directly visualized. A biopsy to remove a tiny piece of tissue can be taken through the endoscope to be examined under the microscope. If a stricture is present, a balloon can be inflated and the area of stricture enlarged or dilated.

This is a very useful procedure for the kinds of problems that scleroderma patients typically have. One difficulty is that it may be hard to pass the endoscope through the mouth in some scleroderma patients due to inability to open the mouth very far. To get around this problem, a pediatric (child-sized) endoscope can be used.

Lower endoscopy or **colonoscopy**: a test in which a tube (colonoscope) is passed through the anus into the rectum and large bowel; this is useful in detecting cancer, polyps, or sources of bleeding in the colon

Sigmoidoscopy: a test in which a tube is passed through the anus only as far as the rectum and part of the colon

Treatment Summary

For reflux: proton pump inhibitor or other ulcer medicine, frequently with a prokinetic agent; reflux precautions include avoiding eating near bedtime, elevating the head of bed, and so on

For decreased motion (decreased peristalsis): prokinetic agent

For bacterial overgrowth and malabsorption: antibiotic or a combination of antibiotics

For constipation: a stool softener on a regular basis, daily or every other day, plus a diet with adequate fiber and a walking exercise program

For watermelon stomach: female hormones, endoscopic cauterization, or removal of part of the stomach

10
✳ ✳ ✳

SCLERODERMA
AND THE LUNGS

Before I begin to discuss how scleroderma can affect the lungs, it is helpful to describe normal lung structure and function. The purpose of the lung is pretty simple: to extract oxygen from the air we breathe (normal room air is 21 percent oxygen) and to get rid of carbon dioxide (CO_2), which is a byproduct of metabolism, the process of converting food products to energy. To do this, the lungs consist of thousands of tiny air sacs (called alveoli), which are arranged around breathing tubes like grapes on a stalk. Air is brought in through the nose and mouth, pulled into the main breathing tube through the voice box, or larynx, and into the trachea, or windpipe (see Figure 2). This divides into the right and left main stem bronchi, large tubes that in turn branch into smaller and smaller air tubes until they reach the smallest tubes, called bronchioles, which have clusters of alveoli around them. The exchange of oxygen for carbon dioxide occurs only in the alveoli. Each

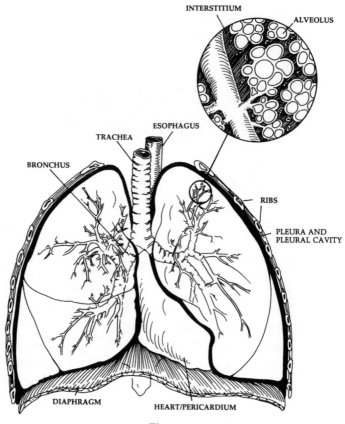

Figure 2

alveolus has a very thin lining or wall composed of a mucous membrane cell on the inside, where the air is, and a capillary (the smallest type of blood vessel) on the outside. Separating the lining cell and the capillary is a very thin structure called a basement membrane, which is made up of collagen.

Blood returning to the heart through the veins passes through the tiny alveolar capillaries one red cell at a time.

Since this is venous blood, the red cell has already lost its oxygen, having given it up to tissues. Oxygen diffuses or passes from the air you breathe into the alveolus across the thin basement membrane into the capillary blood, gets picked up by the hemoglobin in the red cell—hemoglobin is a wonderful molecule with a strong affinity for oxygen; it is also what makes red blood cells red—and gets carried off to the heart for another pass around the circulatory system. As oxygen is diffusing in, carbon dioxide, which is dissolved in the blood serum, passes out of the blood into the air in the alveolus, because the concentration of carbon dioxide in air is much less than in venous blood.

What goes wrong in scleroderma? The basement membrane, between the mucous membrane lining cell and the capillary, is composed of collagen, and scleroderma causes additional collagen to be deposited in this membrane, making it thicker than normal and making it harder and harder for the oxygen to get through into the capillaries. The cell responsible for making this collagen is the pulmonary fibroblast, which resides, along with the mucous membrane lining cell, in the alveolus. Ordinarily the fibroblast doesn't make much collagen; it exists to repair damage from infections, such as pneumonia, or irritation, such as breathing in tiny particles of sand (as, for example, in coal miner's lung disease, or black lung).

What stimulates the fibroblast to make more collagen in scleroderma? There is no apparent infection and no known irritant, so what is going on? We don't know what the initial trigger is, but we do know that there is a cascade of factors coming from activated immune cells and/or damaged blood vessel lining cells, all of which work to activate the fibroblasts.

Alveolitis is the term used to describe the pathological or diseased lung process in scleroderma. This refers to the fact that there is an inflammation in the small air sacs, leading to fibrosis. Sometimes this process goes on slowly and quietly, causing no symptoms until there has been a lot of lung damage. In the early stages, a chest X ray can be normal, but a high-resolution CAT scan of the lungs will be abnormal. Pulmonary function tests are very sensitive in picking up changes in lung function, but they will not distinguish between new fibrosis and old, inactive fibrosis.

Pulmonary fibrosis is the term used to describe the scar tissue buildup in the lungs. Pulmonary fibrosis can be caused by conditions other than scleroderma. These include an inherited form of fibrosis (seen in multiple family members), a reaction to stone dust (seen in miners and sandblasters), or a reaction to some forms of lung inflammation, called adult respiratory distress syndrome (ARDS). These are all fairly unusual occurrences, so the appearance of pulmonary fibrosis on a chest X ray or the development of a restrictive pattern on pulmonary function tests in a scleroderma patient usually means that the fibrosis is due to scleroderma-related lung involvement.

Symptoms

The two major symptoms of pulmonary involvement in scleroderma are coughing and shortness of breath. The cough is usually dry, that is, there is little or no sputum or mucus production. There are several reasons why people can have a chronic or recurrent cough, and there are many reasons for people to be short of breath, so it is necessary to consider all the possibilities before alveolitis can be blamed.

The most common cause of cough in my scleroderma

patients is seasonal allergies, totally unrelated to their scleroderma but very much related to the climate in Michigan,
where I practice. Every spring and every fall, these patients get
a feeling of fullness in the nasal passages and sinuses, and
they experience postnasal drip, hoarseness, cough, and so on.
This also occurs in my lupus and arthritis patients. The point
of this is that not every cough in a scleroderma patient is due
to scleroderma-related lung disease. But if a cough is persistent, lasting more than six weeks, and is not associated with
other signs of allergies, flu, or colds, then a diagnosis of alveolitis should be considered.

The first step in the workup is usually pulmonary function
tests (PFTs), including a diffusion capacity test, which measures the efficiency of gas exchange across the pulmonary
membrane. In this test, people breathe into a machine that
measures airflow and lung volumes. There are three general
patterns of lung abnormalities: asthma, emphysema, and fibrosis. One of the problems in interpreting this test is that in the
early stages of scleroderma-related alveolitis there may be
enough inflammation to evoke a cough response, but there is
not yet enough fibrosis to make the test results very abnormal.
Another complicating factor is lung damage due to smoking.
Such damage will be picked up on the PFTs, confusing the
picture and making the test results more difficult to interpret.
As mentioned above, the chest X ray in the early stages can
also be normal. If this is the case, then a special high-resolution CAT scan of the chest can be done to try to pick up the
"ground glass" appearance of alveolitis in the lung bases. If
this is present, then the diagnosis is firm.

In many situations the picture is not clear-cut, and your
doctor may be concerned that there is an underlying infection
responsible for the cough. If this is the case, the only way to

determine the type of infection is by doing a biopsy, that is, getting a small piece of lung tissue. A biopsy can be done with a bronchoscope, a procedure in which a tube is passed into the lungs and the biopsy taken through the tube. At the time of this procedure, broncho-alveolar lavage (BAL) can also be done through the bronchoscope. In BAL, fluid is passed into one area of the lung and removed by suction. In the removed fluid there are inflammatory cells washed out from the alveoli. These cells can then be analyzed both for the typical pattern of scleroderma and for various infections.

Alternatively, an open biopsy can be done, which is a surgical procedure in which an incision is made in the side of the chest and a piece of lung removed. This yields a larger piece of lung tissue and a better sample.

The bottom line for all of this is that the diagnosis can be unclear. It is essential to make the correct diagnosis, since the treatment of alveolitis is very different from the treatment of an underlying infection and, in fact, might worsen an infection. One or more of these tests may need to be done in order for the diagnosis to be made with certainty. Treatment will be outlined later in this chapter.

Shortness of breath is the other main symptom of scleroderma lung involvement. However, like the development of a cough, it is not specific for alveolitis or fibrosis and can be caused by a number of other things. Shortness of breath, from whatever cause, usually is first noticed with exertion. People complain that they get more winded going up a flight of stairs than they used to. Or they may notice that whereas they used to be able to walk several blocks with ease, now they can walk only one block or have to slow their pace to go more than one block due to shortness of breath. One patient told me that the street in front of his house seemed to have gotten longer.

The main causes of shortness of breath in scleroderma patients are the following: (1) pulmonary fibrosis, (2) deconditioning (being out of shape), (3) a heart problem, (4) muscle weakness due to inflammation (polymyositis) or an underactive thyroid, (5) anemia, or a low red cell count, and (6) pulmonary hypertension. How is all of this sorted out? The chest X ray and pulmonary function tests (PFTs) are helpful, especially if they were done in the previous year or so for comparison. An echocardiogram (ultrasound of the heart) can be very helpful to evaluate heart function and also to test for pulmonary hypertension. Blood tests will help to determine whether there is muscle inflammation, a thyroid problem, or anemia. If the results of all these tests are normal, then the culprit is deconditioning, which is to say that you are out of shape, and the approach is one of physical therapy and exercise.

What if the news is not that good and the diagnosis is alveolitis? What are the treatment options available? Before that question can be answered, I need to distinguish between active inflammation (alveolitis) and established, nonprogressive bibasilar pulmonary fibrosis. Alveolitis should be treated; nonprogressive fibrosis may not need to be.

Treatment of Alveolitis

The treatment of alveolitis is with the medication prednisone and an immunosuppressive medication, usually cyclophosphamide, which is a form of chemotherapy. There is some variation among scleroderma specialists in treatment regimens, particularly in the dose of prednisone and in whether the cyclophosphamide is given as a single intravenous dose on a monthly basis for six to twelve months or as daily pills for the same length of time. However, there is general consensus among treating physicians who see a lot of scleroderma lung disease that this combination of medication is effective in halting or slowing the progression of the lung disease. Other immunosuppressive medications may be useful, such as methotrexate or azathioprine.

The side effects of prednisone (also known as cortisone or glucocorticoid medication) are multiple and can be severe, depending on the dose and the individual's particular reaction. The potential side effects of cyclophosphamide are also serious. This is one of the reasons that physicians like to be very sure about the diagnosis before they recommend this treatment. I will not go into all the potential side effects of these medications here, since I think that this is best discussed between the patient and the doctor on a one-to-one basis. In this situation, the patient has to consider what the alternative to treatment is. If no treatment is given, pulmonary fibrosis will very likely worsen. This can be progressive over a course of several years and can result in pulmonary failure.

Treatment of Nonprogressive Pulmonary Fibrosis

Some individuals have no cough and no shortness of breath, but on physical examination have some abnormal sounds (called rales) when the doctor listens to the lung bases (the bottom of the lungs at the back). A chest X ray may show some scar tissue at the bases, and the PFTs can show a mildly restrictive pattern. A high-resolution CAT scan of the chest may only show the scar tissue and not demonstrate the "ground glass" appearance of inflammation (active alveolitis).

What should be done in this instance? Should prednisone and chemotherapy be given in an attempt to slow down or stop this from getting worse?

The answer depends on the rate of development of the fibrosis. If it is clear that the results of the PFTs have worsened recently and are continuing to worsen, then I think treatment should be initiated. However, I also believe there is time to observe and get a sense of the rapidity of the worsening, especially if there are no recent pulmonary tests that can be used for comparison. In the absence of symptoms (that is, no cough and no shortness of breath), it is reasonable to wait three months and repeat the PFTs, and even to wait another three months and repeat them again. If they are not changing over time, then there is no need to treat. This may be the case when the lung fibrosis is a reaction to reflux, that is, a reaction to small amounts of stomach acid being breathed into the lungs at night. If so, I would recommend antireflux precautions and heartburn medication, as mentioned in the previous chapter.

If, however, there is a slow and gradual decline in the pulmonary function test values, then I think it is very important to treat the problem. There is a difference of opinion regarding how this particular problem should best be approached. Some doctors would use D-penicillamine in this situation, but there is no strong evidence suggesting that one type of treatment is clearly superior to another. This is one of those situations in which more research is needed. I hope in subsequent editions of this book to be able to provide better advice.

In very extreme cases, a lung transplant can be considered. However, the availability of lungs for transplant is low, and there is concern that fibrosis will occur in the transplanted lung as well. These factors have kept transplantation from being a viable option for most scleroderma patients.

Pulmonary Hypertension

Isolated pulmonary hypertension (high blood pressure in the lungs) is a different type of complication that occurs in about 15 percent of scleroderma patients. It can occur with very normal, or even low, systemic blood pressure as measured in the arm. In order to understand this, it is necessary once again to review some anatomy regarding the circulation of blood. Blood leaves the left side of the heart, goes into the arteries, and supplies oxygen to the body. In the process it picks up carbon dioxide and returns via the veins to the right side of the heart. The right side of the heart then pumps it into the lungs through the pulmonary artery. In the lungs, the venous blood gets rid of the carbon dioxide, picks up oxygen, and goes to the left side of the heart to be pumped out to the body again as arterial blood.

Arterial blood is oxygenated and appears bright red; venous blood has lost most of its oxygen and appears dark red or bluish. Arterial blood is under higher pressure than venous blood, so if you puncture an artery, it squirts with every heartbeat. If you puncture a vein, it just oozes blood. Most arteries are buried deeper than veins, to protect them. When you get blood drawn, the technician pokes a vein. However, to get arterial blood gases, or ABGs, for an accurate measurement of the total oxygen in the blood, an artery has to be punctured, and pressure has to be applied for several minutes afterward to stop the bleeding. Rather than get blood gases, I frequently order an oxygen saturation measurement by ear oximetry, which can be done without a needle stick. The information obtained is somewhat different from that given by the ABGs, but the oximetry can be done easily before and after exercise, which is a valuable comparison in individuals who complain about shortness of breath on exertion.

Back to pulmonary hypertension. The pressure in the pulmonary artery needs to be just high enough to push the blood through the lungs. This requires less pressure than that needed to push the blood through the rest of the body. There are two things that can raise pulmonary pressure. One is the loss of volume capacity of the lung vessels. This means that with every heartbeat, the right ventricle (the pumping chamber on the right side) has to try to push the same volume of blood into a smaller volume of space, causing a rise in pressure. This loss of volume capacity happens in extensive pulmonary fibrosis because the capillaries end up "choked off" and can no longer carry as much blood. Another example of loss of volume capacity is when a lung is surgically removed, for example in lung cancer surgery.

However, there is a particular kind of pulmonary hypertension that occurs in the absence of extensive fibrosis and for no apparent reason. This is referred to as isolated pulmonary hypertension and results from a loss of elasticity of the pulmonary artery which becomes narrowed. The right ventricle is trying to pump the same volume of blood into a smaller-diameter tube, so the pressure has to go up. An analogy is a garden hose with an adjustable nozzle. With the nozzle wide open, the pressure is pretty low. As you adjust the nozzle down to a smaller opening, the pressure becomes higher.

What causes this narrowing of the pulmonary artery? And what are the consequences of the higher pressure? I'll answer the second question first. The pumping chamber of the right side of the heart is not made to generate a lot of force. At first it can accommodate a small reduction in the lungs' volume capacity, but as the volume capacity falls, the heart cannot generate enough force to push all of the blood it receives into the lungs. So fluid will back up in the venous system, causing liver congestion and swelling in the lower extremities. This is known as right-sided heart failure.

The answer to the first question of what causes the narrowing is harder to explain. The muscle layer of the artery gets larger, and the inside lining of the artery also gets thicker. The stimulus for all this is not clear.

In terms of diagnosing isolated pulmonary hypertension in scleroderma patients, the best test is an echocardiogram with special attention to the right side of the heart. If this clearly shows that the structures on the right side of the heart are normal, then it is highly unlikely that a significant degree of pulmonary hypertension is present. If the results are abnormal, however, a cardiac catheterization may be done to more precisely measure the right-sided pressures.

In any event, what can be done about this? There are several approaches to treatment. Giving oxygen at night helps, since oxygen serves to relax the smooth muscle of the pulmonary artery. Unfortunately, most blood pressure medicines that work quite nicely for systemic hypertension (the more common type of hypertension, measured by taking the arm blood pressure) have little effect on pulmonary circulation. There is a new class of medicines (called prostacyclin analogues) that are being tested for this condition. One has been shown to be helpful in primary pulmonary hypertension (that is, pulmonary hypertension by itself, without scleroderma) and is currently in clinical trials in scleroderma patients. The problem is that it must be given intravenously, since it does not work in pill form, and it must be given for the rest of the person's life. However, when compared to heart failure, continuous IV treatment may not seem so bad.

Summary of Treatment for
Alveolitis/Pulmonary Fibrosis

1. Stop smoking! Although scleroderma-related lung disease is different from that caused by tobacco, smoking will only make the lung process worse and will also make Raynaud's phenomenon worse.

2. Use measures to prevent gastroesophageal reflux (GERD): elevate the head of the bed, no eating within two hours of bedtime, take medication to treat heartburn, and so on (see Chapter 6).

3. If alveolitis or progressive pulmonary fibrosis is present, an immunosuppressive medication with or without prednisone should be used.

4. If nonprogressive pulmonary fibrosis is present, observe closely with periodic pulmonary function tests.

5. If severe fibrosis is present, home oxygen therapy may be needed.

Summary of Treatment for
Isolated Pulmonary Hypertension

1. Oxygen treatment at night, and occasionally during the day with activity.
2. Intravenous prostacyclin analogues, if severe.

11

* * *

SCLERODERMA AND THE HEART

Scleroderma can affect the heart in several ways. In some cases, heart rhythm can be affected. This is demonstrated by a slow or irregular heartbeat or by an abnormality that is seen only on an electrocardiogram (EKG or ECG). In these cases, the approach to treatment involves either medication to help keep the heartbeat regular or a pacemaker to override the natural electrical system that controls the heartbeat.

Heart rhythm is controlled by an electrical conduction system comprised of specialized cells that generate an electrical current to stimulate the heart muscle to contract in a smooth and regular way. There is a complex system of reflexes that tells the heart to speed up (as with exercise) and to slow down (as with rest), but there is only one electrical system that sends signals to both sides of the heart so that all four chambers contract or pump in a synchronized fashion. The problem that occurs in some cases of scleroderma is that scar tissue (the same culprit we have discussed in the previous chapters) is deposited in the path of the electrical current, so the current is interrupted or blocked. This can be partial or a complete block depending on exactly where it is and how much scar tissue is present. Sometimes the irregular heartbeat is noticed by the patient and sometimes not. It is important to get an EKG to determine exactly what type of problem exists. If no irregularity is picked up on the EKG, then a portable Holter monitor can be given to the patient, which records the EKG for an entire day. This test can pick up heart irregularities that occur only occasionally and are not captured during the short period of time that the EKG is recorded.

Normal heart rhythm is called normal sinus rhythm, since the source of the electrical current comes from a structure in the heart called the sinus node. Changes from normal rhythms are called arrhythmias. There are different terms to describe the dozen or so possible different types of arrhythmias. There is a conduction abnormality called a right bundle branch block, which means that the signal to the right side of the heart is impaired, and (as you would expect) there is a condition known as a left bundle branch block, affecting the left side; then there is a complete heart block. The complete heart block is not as lethal as it sounds, since there is a backup system that permits the heart to beat at a very slow rate (35–40 beats per minute, as opposed to the usual resting heart rate of 60–90 beats per minute) in the absence of sinus node activity. This is not a good situation for the long term, however, and a pacemaker is usually used in the case of complete heart block. There are several other types of cardiac arrhythmias that can happen, some of which make the heat beat too fast rather than too slowly. Some of these arrhythmias need to be treated with either medication or a pacemaker, while others do not.

There are conditions other than scleroderma that can cause conduction problems and arrythmias. The most common of these conditions is coronary artery disease caused by cholesterol buildup; this is the main cause of heart attacks. Just because someone has scleroderma doesn't mean that they cannot get "regular" heart problems. Because of this, a cardiac catheterization may be done. If the diagnosis is usual coronary artery disease, then bypass surgery may be helpful in order to prevent a heart attack.

Another way that scleroderma can affect the heart happens when scar tissue is deposited throughout the heart muscle, not limited to the conduction system, making it a less effective pump. In this case, medication such as digitalis can be helpful. Since, as mentioned above, there are other reasons why someone can have this type of problem, tests such as an echocardiogram as well as an EKG and possibly a stress test and a cardiac catheterization may need to be done to get a good picture of what is going on in a particular case and what is the best approach to treatment.

The third way that scleroderma can affect the heart is by causing inflammation in the outside membrane of the heart, which is called *pericarditis*. The pericardium is a sac that surrounds the heart. When the sac becomes inflamed, fluid accumulates. Sometimes this causes symptoms such as chest pain or shortness of breath, and sometimes it is discovered accidentally by your doctor during a visit for something else. Again, the way to make the diagnosis is by an echocardiogram. If there is a small amount of fluid that does not compress the heart and therefore does not interfere with heart function, medication can be used to treat the inflammation. Typically these medications are either steroids, such as prednisone, or nonsteroidal anti-inflammatory drugs (NSAIDs), such as arthritis medications. If the amount of fluid is very small and there are no symptoms, it is okay to do nothing. If, on the other hand, the fluid volume is quite large and pressing against the heart, compromising the ability of the heart to fill, then a surgical procedure called a pericardial window may need to be done. This permits the fluid to drain out into the lung cavity, where there is more space to accommodate it. Following this, the medication mentioned above can be given to resolve the inflammation over a period of a few weeks. The excess fluid eventually gets reabsorbed back into the bloodstream. Pericarditis is a temporary phenomenon. Although it may recur months or years later, it will resolve again after treatment.

Summary of Heart Involvement

1. Arrythmias are problems with heart rhythm that can be treated with medication or a pacemaker.

2. Heart failure is the inability of the heart chamber to pump out as much blood as is received; this is a problem with heart muscle function that is usually treated with medication.

3. Pericarditis is an inflammation of the sac that surrounds the heart and is treated either with medication or with a surgical procedure called placement of a pericardial window.

Summary of Tests

1. **EKG:** an electrocardiogram, the heart tracing done in a doctor's office that measures heart rate and rhythm

2. **Holter monitor:** a portable EKG monitor usually worn for twenty-four hours to pick up heart rhythm irregularities that may be present only occasionally and that were not picked up by the usual EKG

3. **Echocardiogram:** an ultrasound test of the heart that measures heart function: how well the chambers of the heart are pumping, how well the heart valves are working, and if there is any excess fluid in the sac around the heart

4. **Cardiac catheterization:** a test in which a plastic tube is inserted into a large blood vessel, usually in the groin or in the arm, and threaded into the heart. Contrast material, or IV "dye," is injected into the heart or into the coronary arteries that supply blood to the heart muscle to determine if any vessels are blocked by cholesterol plaques. This procedure can also measure pressures in the heart and in the pulmonary artery to determine if pulmonary hypertension is present.

5. **Cardiac stress test:** a test that determines if the heart is getting an adequate blood supply during exercise. Sometimes the heart will appear normal at rest, and it is only with stress that an abnormality can be demonstrated.

6. **Heart attack or myocardial infarction:** damage to some of the heart muscle due to lack of blood supply from blockage of a coronary artery or due to some severe stress such as malignant phase hypertension (not pulmonary hypertension). Heart attacks are not caused by scleroderma unless there is an episode of malignant phase hypertension (see Chapter 8, on scleroderma and the kidneys).

12

* * *

SCLERODERMA AND JOINTS, TENDONS, MUSCLES, AND NERVES

Stiffness and achiness are common problems in scleroderma. Sometimes patients can't tell whether the aching is
coming from the joints, the muscles, both, or neither. The
thickness and tightness of the overlying skin can make it hard
even for the doctor to determine if joint swelling is present.
This can be an important distinction to make, since joint pain
and swelling (arthritis) may require different treatment than
muscle aches or tendon inflammation. A small percentage of
patients will have a true overlap between rheumatoid arthritis
and scleroderma and may need to be treated with medications
that are usually considered to be specific for rheumatoid
arthritis. Most, however, will not have this overlap.

Joint Stiffness and Arthritis

Many scleroderma patients have hand stiffness that is most
marked in the morning, may or may not be associated with

swelling, and improves with motion during the day. The swelling is not confined to the joints or knuckles of the hands but involves the whole fingers and sometimes the back of the hands as well. The entire hand seems "puffy." The patient cannot make a tight fist, a result of the excess fluid that also causes the puffiness. Many women compare it to fluid retention that commonly occurs just before the menstrual period. This is known as the edematous phase of scleroderma. It is not arthritis; the puffiness is due to damage to small blood vessels that make them leaky, so that excess fluid accumulates in the fingers and hands. This is seldom improved with diuretics, or "water pills," since the underlying problem is not fluid imbalance but damaged blood vessels. This edematous phase can last anywhere from weeks to years but does tend to improve on its own. Frequently it is replaced by a more lasting phase characterized by thickened and tightened skin that causes the fingers to curl down.

True joint stiffness is caused by inflammation in the joints. This can happen in scleroderma patients and is characterized by stiffness in many joints, including the hands, wrists, elbows, shoulders, knees, and ankles. There may or may not be noticeable swelling. The stiffness is worse on waking up and is improved by activity but can recur during the day after periods of inactivity such as riding in a car or sitting in a doctor's waiting room. In order to diagnose the problem, I often ask people if they are stiff when they first get up, and, if so, how long this morning stiffness lasts. (The phenomenon of sitting down and stiffening up again doesn't count in this determination.)

Osteoarthritis (the most common form of arthritis, affecting almost everyone as they get older) is characterized by morning stiffness lasting less than thirty minutes and frequently less than ten minutes. Inflammatory arthritis (such as rheumatoid arthritis and the mildly inflammatory arthritis that accompanies scleroderma and lupus) is characterized by morning stiffness lasting longer than thirty minutes, sometimes several hours. Inflammatory arthritis can be treated with several different types of medication, including the nonsteroidal anti-inflammatory drugs (NSAIDs). One of the potential side effects of this type of medicine is stomach irritation, which can be a problem in individuals already prone to GI upset.

Joint Contractures

Each joint has a normal range of motion, that is, it can be flexed inward, extended outward, or rotated. The elbow, for example, can be extended out straight to 180 degrees and flexed or bent in to about 30 degrees. It can't go any farther because the muscle tissue of the forearm hits the muscle tissue of the upper arm. Contracture of a joint means that the joint cannot be fully flexed or extended; it has lost some of its range of motion. When this occurs due to several different processes, the joints usually develop flexion contractures, in which the joint will not extend fully.

In scleroderma, the fingers tend to be flexed inward and the wrists tend to lose motion in both directions. The elbows may not straighten out fully, and the shoulders can lose motion, so the arms cannot be extended through the normal arc of motion. Maintaining motion may require exercises on a daily basis to keep as much mobility as possible.

Tendonitis and Tendon Rubs

A tendon is a fibrous cord that attaches a muscle to a bone. Tendons are enclosed in a tendon sheath that contains a small amount of fluid to provide for smooth gliding motion. A bursa is a small fluid-filled sac that overlies bony prominences. Tendonitis and bursitis are common problems in the general population, as evidenced by the following nicknames for these conditions: tennis elbow (inflammation of a tendon at the bony protuberance known as the medial epicondyle of the elbow; the condition is also called medial epicondylitis), housemaid's knee (inflammation of the bursa, a padlike sac containing fluid, over the kneecap, also known as prepatellar bursitis), and weaver's bottom (inflammation of the bursa over the "sit-bones," also known as ischial bursitis). However, scleroderma patients get a form of tendonitis that is not usually seen in the general population. The term *tendon rub* describes a sound like two pieces of leather rubbing together; this occurs when a tendon moves in an inflamed, roughened tendon sheath. This happens most commonly at the elbows, the knees, and the ankles. The condition is annoying rather than crippling. The treatment involves applying heat, taking an NSAID medication, and occasional injection of steroids of the area.

Muscles: Polymyositis and Myopathy

Some scleroderma patients have a persistently abnormal elevation in the blood of a muscle enzyme, creatine phosphokinase (CPK), in the blood. This substance comes from the breakdown of muscle, and higher-than-normal levels in the blood imply that muscle is breaking down at a faster-than-normal rate. (Some muscle tissue always breaks down and new muscle is made as part of the body's dynamic equilibrium, so a low level of CPK in the blood is normal.)

There is another autoimmune connective tissue disease known as polymyositis or dermatomyositis (polymyositis accompanied by a particular type of skin rash), which can be seen as an overlap with scleroderma. Symptoms include muscle weakness in the shoulder area and thighs. Although many scleroderma patients will have a sense of overall weakness and fatigue, this condition is distinct. The weakness is usually painless, and people may ignore it at first. In polymyositis, the CPK level in the blood is extremely elevated, sometimes ten times normal. Another muscle enzyme, aldolase, may also be abnormally high. Without treatment, the muscle inflammation can progress to cause destruction of muscles; in very extreme cases it can affect the muscles needed for breathing. It is important to treat this form of polymyositis with medication, usually steroids (cortisonelike medication) alone or steroids plus other immunosuppressive drugs (such as methotrexate or azathioprine). A muscle biopsy may be needed to confirm the diagnosis. This condition tends to have periods of exacerbation and remission, requiring treatment for several months to control the disease, after which the treatment can be stopped for a period of time up to months or years.

The other muscle problem that can occur with scleroderma is nonprogressive scleroderma myopathy. The CPK level in the blood is only modestly elevated (in the range of two to three times normal), and there is little or no muscle weakness. This condition does not affect the respiratory muscles and does not need medication. A muscle biopsy may show that collagen has replaced some muscle fibers, but there is little or no inflammation.

Nerves

Nerve or neurological involvement in scleroderma comes in several different forms. These include entrapment neuropathies, cranial neuropathies, and peripheral sensorimotor neuropathies.

Entrapment neuropathies

Entrapment neuropathies occur when there is pressure put on a nerve, causing either pain or a tingling kind of numbness in the area that is supplied by the nerve. The most common form of entrapment neuropathy in the general population and in scleroderma patients is carpal tunnel syndrome. One of the major nerves to the hands is called the median nerve and goes through a narrow tunnel (the carpal tunnel) at the base of the palm. If this area becomes narrowed, by swelling from wrist arthritis, tendonitis, or other causes, pain or numbness will occur. This happens a lot in pregnant women, who tend to have swelling in both hands and feet; fortunately, it usually resolves spontaneously after delivery. Diabetics are prone to get this, too, as are people with rheumatoid arthritis involving the wrists. Scleroderma patients get it due to the swelling from leaking blood vessels, mentioned above, or from scar tissue buildup. The symptoms are numbness and tingling in the thumb, index, and long fingers, which tends to be worse at night and can awaken people from sleep. Sometimes it is difficult to distinguish between the tingling from

Raynaud's phenomenon and the tingling from carpal tunnel syndrome. The usual way to figure this out is that Raynaud's tingling happens in response to cold exposure, and carpal-tunnel-related tingling happens when there is no change in temperature.

Other nerves can get trapped as well. The ulnar nerve, the nerve that is responsible for the "funny bone" feeling when you hit your elbow and get a painful shock that travels down into the little finger, gets very close to the skin surface when it goes around the elbow. In scleroderma the skin can get very tight at the elbow, the tendons shorten, and the elbow cannot be straightened out all the way. Sometimes the tightness is so severe that it presses on the nerve and causes pain down the forearm and into the little finger.

What can be done about entrapment neuropathies? For carpal tunnel syndrome or median nerve compression, wrist splints are recommended to hold the wrist and hand in the best position to open up the narrowed tunnel. Cortisone injections are sometimes used to relieve the inflammation that the pressure causes. In severe circumstances, surgery can be performed to open up the tunnel. Surgery can be done for ulnar neuropathy (at the elbow), but it is less successful than the carpal tunnel surgery and so should be approached with caution.

Cranial neuropathies

The cranial nerves are those that go to the head and are responsible for moving the muscles of the face and eyes and for providing sensation to these areas. Problems with these nerves are more often seen in lupus but can also occur in scleroderma. Occasionally scleroderma can cause a condition called Bell's palsy, which results in a droop of the face on one side. Bell's palsy can be caused by many different conditions (sometimes a virus) and may respond to prednisone (also known as cortisone) treatment.

Scleroderma can be associated with a painful condition called trigeminal neuralgia, or tic douloureux (meaning "painful spasm"). This is caused by inflammation of the nerve that is responsible for providing sensation to one side of the face. When this nerve becomes inflamed, it causes pain that can wax and wane in intensity, sometimes being sharp and sometimes causing a pins-and-needles or numb sensation. If this condition does not respond to medication, does not resolve on its own, and is very severe, the nerve may need to be surgically cut. This leaves an area of the face permanently numb, but numbness may be preferable to persistent or recurrent pain.

Peripheral sensorimotor neuropathies

Sometimes nerves in other areas of the body will be affected, leading to numbness or tingling in a pattern that is different from the carpal tunnel syndrome or ulnar nerve problems noted in the section on entrapment neuropathies. Occasionally there will also be weakness of a muscle leading to a foot drop, that is, the inability to pick up the toes when walking. This is usually due to vasculitis, inflammation of a blood vessel that supplies nutrition to a nerve. Without the blood supply, the nerve weakens and dies. The diagnosis is usually made based on the patient's symptoms. Since the underlying problem is an inflammation, the treatment is medication such as steroids (cortisone or prednisone) or other immunosuppressive medications. The nonsteroidal anti-inflammatory medicines (NSAIDs) are usually not strong enough to be helpful in this situation.

Fibrositis or Fibromyalgia

Some scleroderma patients are also bothered with fibrositis or fibromyalgia. These two terms refer to a painful condition characterized by tender areas, called trigger points, at the base of the neck, across the upper back and shoulders, the low back, the inside of the knees, and the inside of the elbows. Fibromyalgia is associated with poor sleep patterns and sometimes with depression or anxiety. It is not clear if the pain starts first and then interferes with sleep or if the abnormal sleep pattern comes first and causes the muscle tenderness, but what is clear is that the pain and poor sleep go hand in hand.

Fibromyalgia is a very common condition in the general population, affecting people of all age groups. The treatment is usually a combination of physical therapy along with medication to improve sleep patterns or to relieve depression.

Physical Therapy

The role of physical therapy in the treatment of scleroderma varies from one person to the next. Most individuals benefit from a program that teaches them about range-of-motion exercises they can do in their own home. Muscles that do not move will weaken and shrink (atrophy). The difficult part (as with all exercise programs) is to maintain a schedule of regular exercise for the long term.

As mentioned above, wrist splints can help with symptoms of carpal tunnel syndrome, and hand splints, used at night, may be useful to prevent or slow down flexion contractures of the fingers. Inflammatory arthritis of the hand joints may be helped by heat treatments, such as hot wax baths, but these should not be used if finger sores are present.

An exercise program has more benefits than just increased strength, improved mobility, and longer endurance. Exercise improves mood, helps restore normal sleep patterns, and results in a better sense of well-being and independence.

Some people get discouraged because they can no longer perform at the level they were at prior to their illness. Just because you cannot run marathons does not mean you cannot walk daily, ride an exercise bike, or participate in a pool exercise program. For example, the Arthritis Foundation (with chapters in all fifty states) offers exercise programs at community and private indoor pools throughout the country, and there are many other programs available.

13

* * *

SYSTEMIC SCLERODERMA
AND PREGNANCY

Young women with systemic scleroderma often ask me if it is okay to get pregnant. The answer is that it depends on several factors: the stage of the disease, the medications that are required to control the disease, and the risks that people are willing to take in order to have a child. (Note that this does not apply to people with localized scleroderma, a condition that does not present a higher-than-usual risk during pregnancy. However, the use of any medication needs to be reviewed by the patient and her doctor before pregnancy occurs.)

Pregnancy is a strain on the body even for individuals who are otherwise well. Even a normal pregnancy in a healthy individual can be complicated by high blood pressure, diabetes, kidney problems, circulation problems, heartburn, hemorrhoids, and a host of other difficulties. Pregnancy in a scleroderma patient has particular problems and is considered a high-risk condition, requiring careful monitoring of the mother and the baby. Many of my patients have successfully gotten pregnant, had a medically uneventful course, and delivered healthy babies. Others have not been this fortunate. Pregnancy has different effects on people with different connective tissue diseases. For example, in most cases pregnancy makes rheumatoid arthritis *better* and lupus *worse*. There does not seem to be a consistent effect on scleroderma patients; some do quite well and others do not.

It is important to consider the risks before contemplating pregnancy. If a patient has been diagnosed recently, I suggest that she wait to get pregnant for at least two or three years, to get a better idea of what type of scleroderma she has. Limited scleroderma presents less risk than diffuse disease, although there is some increase in blood pressure and risk of kidney problems in both types. People with diffuse disease run a greater risk of blood pressure problems, kidney disease, and heart disease.

Problems for the baby that can occur in scleroderma pregnancies include stillbirth, miscarriages, and low birth weight. Problems for the mother include serious blood pressure problems with the risk of kidney failure, strokes, and heart problems. There is a condition called preeclampsia that can occur in the absence of scleroderma but is somewhat more common in scleroderma patients. This condition is characterized by severe high blood pressure, swelling of the legs, and kidney damage. If preeclampsia is left untreated, it can progress to eclampsia, which causes seizures and is associated with a high mortality for both mothers and babies. The main treatment for preeclampsia is to deliver the baby, even though premature. In scleroderma the source of the problem is damage to the blood vessels in the placenta, which is the sac that surrounds the baby, provides it with nutrition and oxygen, and removes wastes. In this disease these blood vessels become thickened and narrowed, much like blood vessels elsewhere in the body.

The decision whether to have a child is a serious one that should be made after gathering information and discussing it with your loved ones, as there are several issues involved.

Getting Pregnant

Women with scleroderma, like all women with a chronic disease, may have a harder time getting pregnant than their healthier counterparts. Menstrual abnormalities or irregular periods may be a sign that ovulation (the production of eggs) may not be occurring in a normal fashion. It is generally true, not just for scleroderma patients, that the longer one waits to become pregnant, the more difficult it can be to conceive.

Very little is known about the risks of using fertility drugs in people who have scleroderma. Since 80 percent of scleroderma patients are female, and since it is thought that female (estrogen-type) hormones play some role in the susceptibility to scleroderma (see Chapter 6), fertility drugs may be dangerous in scleroderma patients since they induce a high-estrogen state.

Also, some medications used for scleroderma can contribute to infertility. Drugs such as prednisone (a form of cortisone) can cause menstrual irregularities and decreased fertility. Other medicines such as cyclophosphamide can contribute to the onset of early menopause. Certain medications may not affect a woman's ability to get pregnant but could cause damage to the fetus (the developing baby) if they were taken during pregnancy. This is why it is very important to consult with your doctor about your desire to have a baby *before* you actually get pregnant. Most medications would have to be stopped before it would be safe to conceive a child.

Because of this requirement to stop medications, it is important that the scleroderma be stable, with no evidence of high blood pressure or active pulmonary disease, before getting pregnant. Women with preexisting heart muscle dysfunction should probably avoid pregnancy. Women with some forms of heart conduction defects (a blocked heart rhythm) may still safely get pregnant, as long as the heart rhythm can be controlled by a pacemaker. Medications to prevent reflux (heartburn) need to be stopped as well. This may mean worse heartburn, but antacids can be safely substituted. Each patient is different.

The Course of Pregnancy

Pregnancy in a scleroderma patient should always be considered high-risk and followed by an obstetrician familiar with such high-risk situations, in collaboration with the treating rheumatologist. Ideally medications will have been stopped before the pregnancy occurred. Certainly once a woman is pregnant, the usual scleroderma medications have to be stopped in order to prevent problems for the baby.

The normal nausea or morning sickness in early pregnancy can be exaggerated in some scleroderma patients. Individuals need to check their blood pressure frequently, twice a week or more often, to make sure that it stays under good control. If the blood pressure goes up, medication needs to be given to lower it. There are some medicines that are safer during pregnancy than others, and the usual type of medicine to lower scleroderma-related high blood pressure, an ACE inhibitor (mentioned in Chapter 8, Scleroderma and the Kidneys), is not given unless other medicines cannot adequately manage the situation.

If severe hypertension (preeclampsia) occurs and the

blood pressure cannot be adequately controlled by medication, then the baby needs to be delivered, usually by cesarean section and regardless of the degree of prematurity. This is the most dangerous complication for scleroderma patients and for the baby. This is one of those "what if" situations that the patient, along with her family and her doctor, needs to address prior to or early in the course of the pregnancy. It can be a difficult and sad situation, but individuals need to weigh the risks and benefits and decide what is best for them.

Heartburn is a common and almost universal symptom in pregnancy, even for those without scleroderma, so it is easy to understand that it will be especially pronounced in those with the disease. The proton pump inhibitors are *not* usually given in pregnancy, making this problem extra difficult. Antireflux measures such as elevating the head of the bed, avoiding eating in the two hours before bedtime, avoiding caffeine, and using antacids are helpful.

Is there any good news in all of this? Well, actually there is. Raynaud's phenomenon usually improves in pregnancy. A small point, perhaps, but most people enjoy this.

Labor and Delivery

For the most part, once the pregnancy has reached term, labor and delivery are no different for the scleroderma patient than for anyone else.

Case Histories

One of my patients, now in her mid-twenties, has had systemic scleroderma from the age of eleven. She was quite sick in the first few years and had malignant phase hypertension and kidney problems, all of which were treated promptly. She recovered 90 percent of her kidney function. Her skin has returned almost totally to normal in terms of skin thickness and tightness, but she has quite a few telangiectasias (red spots) on her face, arms, legs, and trunk. She still has some reflux symptoms and has Raynaud's attacks. Her blood pressure "acts up" about twice a year, requiring treatment with an ACE inhibitor for a few months. She has no evidence of heart or lung involvement. She wanted to get pregnant, so I advised her to stop her medication first and see how things went for a few months. All was well, so she went ahead and got pregnant.

Just a few weeks ago she was in my office to show off the baby, now ten months old. She had problems during her pregnancy with blood pressure, which was treated successfully with no damage to her kidneys. She had a cesarean section (probably unrelated to the scleroderma) at the end of a full-term pregnancy and is doing just fine.

Not everyone is so lucky. Another patient, in her early thirties, had systemic scleroderma for six years. By all measures the disease was stable, with no development of new heart, lung, blood pressure, or kidney problems for about two years. She and her husband were both eager to have children. Late in the second trimester, at about six months, she developed malignant phase hypertension that could not be controlled, and she went into kidney failure and lost the baby. She is now on dialysis, some four years later, and is considering a kidney transplant. She and her husband have since adopted a child.

Another of my patients, with both diffuse scleroderma and rheumatoid arthritis, decided to adopt rather than run the risk of a pregnancy.

Many scleroderma patients successfully get pregnant, have healthy babies, and do very well. Other individuals decide to forgo pregnancy because of the risk of damaging their own health and losing the baby. Every case is different, and it is an individual decision. Parenthood is one of the greatest joys in life and also one of the greatest responsibilities. Although the facts presented in this chapter may be sobering, there is no right decision for all. Any decision, however, should be an informed one.

14

* * *

SCLERODERMA
AND
SEXUALITY

Sexuality involves the physiological and the psychological, the body and the mind. These two features are always intertwined in human behavior, but they are particularly so in the realm of sexuality. This chapter is divided into three sections: on women, on men, and on spouses.

Women, Scleroderma, and Sexuality

Physical problems for women with scleroderma include fatigue, dryness of the vagina (as part of Sjogren's syndrome), and physical discomfort during sex that is a result of decreased mobility of joints, sometimes associated with joint pain. Also, symptoms of reflux (heartburn) can be worsened by lying flat and by having the weight of a body on top.

Fatigue

Fatigue is a common problem in the general population. Sometimes it is difficult to distinguish the fatigue that is associated with depression or hopelessness from the fatigue that commonly accompanies a connective tissue disease. My patients frequently tell me that it is all they can do to go to work each day, much less have extra energy to devote to their families in the evening. What frequently goes unstated is that this level of fatigue also means there is not enough energy to enjoy an active sexual relationship with their partner. Women seldom bring this up. Fatigue is considered a personal problem, a fault, a failing. Fatigued people are thought of as "lazy" or simply as lacking the motivation to get things done.

Also, fatigue tends to develop gradually and is sometimes unnoticed until either medication is given or the disease begins to stabilize. Patients will then comment to me that they are feeling better and suddenly have their energy back again.

From a doctor's point of view, fatigue is a difficult symptom to treat. There is no medication that will magically make it go away and restore energy. My advice is to stop beating yourself up over it. I have a patient who tells me that she has a Plan A and a Plan B. Plan A is for the days when her energy level is high. In addition to her necessary activities, she can take on some extra projects. Plan B is for the days when she knows she has to take it easy. She considers Plan B days as those for rest and restoration. She has had more Plan A days than Plan B days over the course of her illness, but she tries to avoid labeling them as "good days" and "bad days." Both are part of the ebb and flow of her life now. She is fortunate in having an understanding family who are keyed into the plans. If there is a special outing scheduled, she rests up to prepare herself for it. This outlook on life requires the confidence that there will be Plan A days and the acceptance that Plan B days happen and are okay.

I wish I could take this attitude and transplant it into others. But too often it happens that constant fatigue can nudge people into depression. Fatigue and depression are closely interrelated—fatigue can lead to depression, just as depression is usually associated with fatigue. A patient whom I saw recently was complaining bitterly about her fatigue. She has five-year-old twins, as well as two school-age children. She had to quit her job due to her fatigue. Even without working outside the home, she was still tired a great deal. I tried to point out to her that just being home with her children was a gift to them, but she didn't buy it. She complained that her older children sometimes had to help her out with the younger ones. I said it would teach them responsibility, but she was stuck. All she could see was her shortcomings. She was unable to get pleasure from what she *was* able to do.

This is a common feature of depression. Depressed individuals are unable to see the whole picture. They are blocked from enjoyment, and no amount of arguing will convince them otherwise. Persistent depression like this may require professional help.

If sex is important to your relationship (as it usually is), then resting up for it or planning for it may become necessary. Although this may take away some of the spontaneity, the rewards of having an active sex life will make up for this.

Vaginal Dryness

Sjogren's syndrome frequently accompanies systemic scleroderma. This causes dryness of the mucous membranes, typically leading to symptoms of dry eyes and dry mouth. The vagina can also become dry, with less lubrication during arousal, making sex uncomfortable or even painful. Vaginal lubricants that can be purchased in most drugstores are very helpful. However, before you blame scleroderma and Sjogren's syndrome, it is important to realize that vaginal dryness can also occur with menopause and the drop of female hormones that accompanies it. If this is the case, either estrogen replacement hormones in pill form or an estrogen-containing vaginal cream can be useful.

Joint Discomfort

Some women find sex painful because they have trouble finding a comfortable position. Joints are stiff and sore, or limbs just don't move the way they used to. A warm bath may help to loosen up joints. The real resolution to this problem is imagination, creativity, a sense of humor, and a loving partner.

Emotional and Psychological Issues

Emotional and psychological issues also get in the way of sexual enjoyment. These include depression, which typically decreases sex drive; changes in body image, leading to the fear that you are not as attractive as before; and anxiety that sex will be painful. Male partners of women with scleroderma can be affected by this attitude of heightened anxiety and retreat from sex for fear of causing pain and discomfort in the women they love. In the absence of good communication, both partners can fall into a world of silence that fosters isolation and loneliness. This is an area where a counselor can be tremendously helpful. If one of the partners is reluctant to talk about such personal issues in the presence of a "stranger," the other partner can go alone and talk about fears of the illness and what it means for both partners and their future. The real issue is communication, more so than the technical aspects of sexual intercourse. Once communication is reestablished, the rest will follow.

Men, Scleroderma, and Sexuality

I have written several times in this book that 80 percent of scleroderma patients are women. This, obviously, leaves 20 percent that are men. I have seen and treated over five hundred scleroderma patients, which means that I have seen approximately a hundred male patients. The most common complaint I hear from male patients regarding sexual problems involves impotence, particularly the ability to get and maintain an erection. There are several possible explanations for this. These include neurological abnormalities, vascular problems, medication side effects, and psychological and emotional difficulties.

Neurological Abnormalities

The penis becomes erect when more blood is directed into it than is drained from it. This requires the coordinated action of blood vessels and nerves. The part of the nervous system that is responsible for this is called the sympathetic nervous system, which is part of a network that transmits signals from the brain to various parts of the body. There is some evidence from medical research that the sympathetic nervous system can be damaged in scleroderma, and this may account for difficulties with erection in some patients.

Vascular Problems

Vascular problems are common in scleroderma. Damage to blood vessels is what causes Raynaud's phenomenon, finger sores, and high blood pressure. The blood supply to the penis can also be affected.

The key issue is what can be done about it. Unfortunately, once the damage is done to the blood vessels or to the nerves, it may not be possible to reverse it. There is a recently approved medication (sildenafil) that improves the circulation to the penis and can improve erectile function, though there are no long-term studies of its safety and no studies at all in scleroderma patients. I recommend that patients discuss the alternatives with their doctor, who may suggest a consultation with a urologist who is also a specialist in problems of impotence. Besides medication, there are external devices that can be applied to the penis to stimulate an erection; these may work for some people. There are also implantable devices that can be used. The point is that there are treatments for this problem.

Medication Side Effects

Problems with erections can also be the result of side effects from medication. This is occasionally seen with a common medication that is used to treat Raynaud's phenomenon and finger ulcers, namely, nifedipine or other calcium channel blockers. It is paradoxical that medications used to improve the circulation to the fingers can result in impaired circulation to the penis, but this is the case. I would strongly suggest that you discuss the issue with your doctor before stopping the medication and that you get a workup by a urologist.

Psychological and Emotional Difficulties

Psychological and emotional problems also play a key role in sexual function. A decrease in sex drive (libido) commonly occurs with fatigue and depression. Fatigue can be a feature of all connective tissue diseases (rheumatoid arthritis, lupus, and scleroderma). As noted above, some people dismiss the fatigue as "laziness" and think that if they just push themselves harder, it will go away. But listen to your body. If it is telling you that you need more rest, then you need more rest.

Depression can also deprive people of the ability to enjoy life, and along with this may come loss of libido. There are many reasons for depression, and none should be dismissed out of hand. Many of my male patients have expressed concern over holding their jobs, and they frequently will not tell their employers of their illness if this is at all possible. Accepting disability or a decreased level of activity is difficult emotionally for many men, especially if it is associated with a loss of income. Some men feel guilty for bringing economic hardship to their families. Wives may resent bearing the burden of supporting the family.

There is another feature of scleroderma that is unique for men. Most of my male patients have told me at one time or another that they resent having a "female" disease. In this culture, men are not supposed to get sick; if sick, they are not supposed to dwell on it. Given this, it may be exceptionally difficult for a man to disclose that he has scleroderma and then hear the response "Oh, I thought that was a woman's disease." But the fact that scleroderma affects mostly women does not mean that a man who has it is less than male. Male hormone levels are normal in scleroderma patients; sperm production is good, and male patients can father children. In other words, there is no apparent defect in "maleness" caused by or related to scleroderma.

One additional problem that can occur with male scleroderma patients is that a band of thickened skin can develop on the side of the penis and interfere with erection and/or make the erect penis crooked. If mild, nothing needs to be done. If severe enough to interfere with intercourse, then a surgical procedure can be done to remove some of this scar tissue and straighten the penis.

Spouses, Scleroderma, and Sexuality

So your spouse has scleroderma. What does this mean for you? It means that life is different from what it used to be. All things of importance that happen to you affect your relationship with your spouse, and the same is true of important things that happen to her or him. Certainly if you changed jobs, decided to become a vegetarian, or converted to a different religion, it would have an impact on your spouse. All of these things profoundly affect your day-to-day activities, your view of the world, and your view of yourself. Getting a rare, incurable, and chronic disease is one of those life-changing events. The difference between this and other life changes is that getting this disease is nonvoluntary. You can *hope* that your spouse will have a mild form of scleroderma, with little impact on usual activities and no impact on longevity, but you can't count on it.

You can call it unfair, and you will be right. You can protest that your life should not have to change, and you will be wrong. If you are too busy, then you will have to let something else go. If you can't handle it alone, then you must get help. You may feel that your spouse is too demanding, is wallowing in self-pity, or is exaggerating symptoms. This may actually be the case. If so, then both of you need to work out your feelings of disappointment, resentment, anger at the disease, or whatever is behind this behavior.

Sometimes the unaffected partner can develop an "Oh, you poor thing! Let me do that for you" attitude toward his or her spouse. But pity takes away responsibility, robs individuals of the means to influence their own lives, and turns them into passive recipients dependent on the goodwill of others. Pity may feel good in the short term, but it is poison in the long term. Just because someone needs help in some areas of living does not mean that they are helpless. Resentment in this situation frequently goes both ways.

Striking a new balance in a relationship is a very difficult thing to do. People get used to their roles and resent change, especially change that is forced upon them by circumstances beyond their control. But change can also be a challenge, an opportunity, a chance to reexamine what is important in life.

I have seen marriages become stronger in the face of this type of adversity. Unfortunately, I have also watched marriages fall apart. In the latter case, it is usually because the relationship was rocky before the onset of illness—communication was poor to begin with, and one or both partners were not committed to making things work. The illness then becomes the excuse for the breakup, but the real reasons go much deeper. Whatever your personal situation, know that you cannot successfully address these issues alone. Turn to your loved ones for support. Get professional help if you need it. If you cannot afford it or if your insurance does not cover this type of service, you can turn to your church or synagogue. Most priests, ministers, or rabbis can offer support or can suggest where such support can be obtained.

15

✳ ✳ ✳

OVERLAP SYNDROMES AND SCLERODERMALIKE CONDITIONS

In most cases, the connective tissue diseases—rheumatoid arthritis, lupus, scleroderma, polymyositis, and dermatomyositis—occur as separate entities. Occasionally, more than one of these diseases will coexist in the same patient, and these people are said to have overlap syndromes, with features of two or more diseases. Sjogren's syndrome is the exception in that it most usually coexists with the above diseases, although there are cases when it occurs alone. Sometimes one connective tissue disease will exist by itself for several years before the features of another condition develop. This tends to cause confusion in people who, having been told that they have one disease, are then told that they have another. Since many symptoms are similar among the conditions, making the diagnosis of one versus another can be difficult, particularly in the early stages.

Mixed Connective
Tissue Disease

Mixed connective tissue disease, or MCTD, is a combination of lupus, scleroderma, and polymyositis along with a positive blood test for an antibody to ribonucleic protein (RNP). RNP is a protein that is attached to RNA, or ribonucleic acid, part of the machinery in the cell for manufacturing proteins from the genetic code of DNA. It is not clear why an antibody is produced to this protein, and it is not clear that this antibody actually plays any role in the development of the disease. There is only the observation that this antibody is seen in association with MCTD and serves as a useful test to help make the diagnosis.

In order to explain this condition, it may be helpful to describe a patient. I first saw one young woman about ten years ago. She had diffuse scleroderma with a lot of skin involvement. At that time her ANA (antinuclear antibody) was positive, as it is in 85 percent of scleroderma patients and in 95 percent of lupus patients. However, she had no features of lupus. Her RNP antibody test was negative. About two years later she developed very severe muscle inflammation (polymyositis) and became so weak she had trouble walking. This inflammation improved with steroids and an immunosuppressive medication, and over the following two years she regained her strength but had problems with lung fibrosis. Two years later she developed fluid around her heart (pericarditis) and was admitted to the hospital to get the fluid drained. She also had vasculitis (inflammation of blood vessels) that produced a wrist drop that was more typical of lupus than of scleroderma. On repeat testing, she was shown to now have RNP antibodies. I saw her in the office recently. She is on home oxygen but her lung function is stable, her heart is fine, and she is walking with a walker.

MCTD can start as scleroderma, as lupus, or as polymyositis. The sequence of events will vary from one person to the next.

Scleroderma and Polymyositis

This is an overlap that occurs in about 25 percent of scleroderma patients. The polymyositis occurs as a gradual, and usually painless, muscle weakness that affects the shoulder muscles and the hip muscles more than the muscles of the hands or feet. The blood levels of muscle enzymes (CPK and aldolase) are increased, and a test of muscle function called an EMG will show evidence of muscle damage. A muscle biopsy may be needed to confirm the diagnosis. Treatment usually consists of steroids and immunosuppressive agents. Frequently this treatment is needed for only one to two years and then can be stopped without recurrence of muscle inflammation.

Scleroderma and Rheumatoid Arthritis

These two diseases coexist in only 5 to 10 percent of scleroderma cases. It is not enough for the blood test for rheumatoid factor to be positive; for there to be a diagnosis of rheumatoid arthritis in conjuction with scleroderma, the physician will need to see X-ray evidence of damage or erosions in the joints.

The treatment is the same as for rheumatoid arthritis without scleroderma.

Scleroderma and Lupus

This is another unusual combination, occurring in about 5 percent of scleroderma cases. I did not think this condition really existed until one of my patients proved me wrong. She is an individual with limited scleroderma that began almost twenty years ago. I have been following her for the last eight years or so. She is doing quite well and continues to work, and I had pretty much stopped worrying about her, seeing her every six months or so. She called one day and told me that her feet were swelling and that she just wasn't feeling very well. I saw her in the office and ordered some tests. To my surprise, she had protein and red cells in her urine and a positive anti-DNA antibody test (a test very specific for lupus). The protein loss in the urine was responsible for her swelling. A kidney biopsy confirmed lupus kidney disease, and she was treated for one year with steroids and immunosuppressives. The protein in her urine cleared up, her kidney function remains normal, and I am back to seeing her every six months.

Scleroderma and Sjogren's Syndrome

This is a common combination. Sjogren's syndrome is characterized by dry mucous membranes, that is dry eyes, dry mouth, and in women a dry vagina. It is caused by an immune attack on the glands that produce mucus and saliva in these organs. Again, it is not known why the immune system becomes activated to recognize this target as foreign.

The lack of tears causes the eyes to feel dry, irritated, and "gritty." There can be dried secretions in the inner corner of the eye on awakening in the morning. If severe, there can be abrasions or ulcers that develop on the cornea, the clear covering over the pupil and iris, and this can eventually interfere with vision.

Lack of saliva causes the mouth to feel dry. However, there are many reasons for a dry mouth other than Sjogren's syndrome. Perhaps the most common cause of mouth dryness is the habit of breathing through the mouth, which occurs in people with allergies or sinus problems. Many medications, including over-the-counter ones, have dry mouth as a side effect. These include antihistamines, decongestants, some blood pressure pills, antidepressant medicines, and numerous others. The problem of decreased production of saliva is not just discomfort. Saliva helps to control the normal bacteria in the mouth and prevent tooth cavities. People with Sjogren's syndrome need to see a dentist more frequently and need to be more careful with brushing and flossing. This can be a difficult problem if the mouth cannot be opened wide due to scleroderma.

Lack of vaginal moisture and lubrication can make sexual intercourse uncomfortable and even painful. This is not always due to Sjogren's but can also occur after menopause, with the loss of estrogen. In some people it may be a combination of both conditions. Estrogen replacement, either by pills, skin patches, or a vaginal cream, can help if the dryness is primarily due to estrogen deficiency. If this is not the case, then vaginal lubrication before sexual activity will be necessary.

Petroleum jelly is *not* recommended. There are many over-the-counter preparations specifically formulated as vaginal lubricants that are very helpful.

Scleroderma and Thyroid Disease: Hashimoto's and Graves' Disease

Thyroid problems can result in an underactive thyroid (Hashimoto's thyroiditis) or an overactive thyroid (Graves' disease). Both of these conditions are caused by an immune attack on the thyroid tissue.

The thyroid gland is located in the front of the neck just below the Adam's apple. It controls the metabolic rate of the entire body. Typical symptoms of an underactive thyroid are weight gain, fatigue, dry skin, and constipation. Symptoms of an overactive thyroid are weight loss, diarrhea, jitteriness, and a fast heart rate. These symptoms can also be seen in scleroderma itself, and often occur in people without thyroid problems. Fortunately, there is a simple blood test that measures thyroid activity.

Scleroderma and Other Diseases

Just because you have scleroderma does not mean that you cannot get other conditions. The above overlap syndromes are particular situations. However, scleroderma patients can still get other common conditions such as colds, flu, bladder infections, and so on. In addition, people with scleroderma still have the same risk as those without scleroderma of developing more serious conditions such as breast cancer or uterine cancer. You still need routine checkups and, for women, Pap smears and breast exams.

Undifferentiated Connective Tissue Disease (UCTD)

Some people experience a few signs and symptoms, and even some laboratory test abnormalities, that suggest they have a connective tissue disease, but the picture is incomplete. They "almost" have lupus or scleroderma, but not quite. They do not fit nicely into the diagnostic categories that the textbooks describe. It is wrong to diagnose such people as having scleroderma or lupus if they do not have these diseases. Rather, they are said to have undifferentiated connective tissue disease, or UCTD. In one study that followed a number of patients for many years, about one third of people with UCTD went on to develop a defined disease (that is, they fulfilled the textbook definition), about one third got better, and about one third stayed in the "gray zone."

Although this may be an unsatisfactory diagnosis for some people, it is about as good as we can get in terms of accurately defining our diseases. In the future, when we find out what actually causes autoimmune diseases, we will be able to specify particular tests and provide a better diagnosis. Until then, UCTD will remain a possible diagnosis.

Sclerodermalike Disorders

There are some conditions that resemble scleroderma but have certain features that are quite distinct. Because of these differences, they are usually classified as sclerodermalike disorders. These include eosinophilic fasciitis, sclerodema or scleromyxedema, chronic graft versus host disease, and eosinophilia myalgia syndrome.

Eosinophilic Fasciitis (EF)

In eosinophilic fasciitis (EF), white blood cells (eosinophils and leukocytes) attack the fascia, which is a thin sheet of tissue that separates muscle from the fat and skin above it. In some cases the fascia becomes inflamed, that is, it becomes swollen and tender. The skin overlying the fascia appears puckered, like the skin of an orange, and the tissue under the skin feels hard (some say that it feels like wood). Eosinophilic fasciitis affects the arms, legs, and trunk while sparing the hands and face, since there is little fascia in the hands and face. Also, contractures of the elbows or knees and decreased range of motion at the shoulders, hips, and central body occur rapidly, within a few weeks of the onset of the skin changes. This is more rapid than with scleroderma. Joint pains and carpal tunnel syndrome are frequently seen, which is also true in systemic scleroderma. Usually (but not always) there is no Raynaud's phenomenon, and the ANA is negative.

The diagnosis of EF is made on the basis of the pattern of skin involvement (for example, if the hands are affected, it cannot be EF; systemic sclerosis, by contrast, *can* affect the hands), on the basis of the appearance of the skin and feel of the tissue, and on a deep biopsy of skin, fat, and fascia. Sometimes a blood test will also show high levels of eosinophils.

The cause of this condition is not known. Eosinophils are a type of white blood cell that are important in allergic reactions and in some autoimmune diseases. A higher-than-normal eosinophil count is seen in some people with scleroderma, both systemic and localized. This does not mean that they are "allergic" to something; at the very least, we don't know what they are allergic to. Eosinophilic fasciitis is sometimes seen after a period of unusually heavy exercise or after significant trauma. In many cases, however, there is no apparent initiating event. Treatment consists of cortisonelike medication and immunosuppressive medications.

Sclerodema or Scleromyxedema

Sclerodema, also known as scleromyxedema, is a condition characterized by thickened skin of the face, head, neck, and shoulders; the thickening can extend down into the arms. Sometimes it affects the trunk as well, though it spares the hands. Usually (but not always) there is no Raynaud's phenomenon, and the ANA is negative.

This condition is usually associated with long-standing diabetes or with a bone marrow abnormality that can be either benign (not cancerous) or malignant (cancerous). If the cause is diabetes, then it is important to get very tight control of the blood sugar. If the cause is a bone marrow abnormality, then treatment of the underlying disease will often improve the symptoms.

Chronic Graft versus Host Disease (GVHD)

Graft versus host disease occurs in a very specific and unusual setting. It happens in some people who get bone marrow transplants as part of treatment for some forms of cancer. High dose chemotherapy is first given to the patient to get rid of the cancer cells. The chemotherapy also results in the destruction of the patient's bone marrow which is responsible for making red cells, white cells, and platelets. Since the white cells are killed off, the patient's immune system is also destroyed.

Following the chemotherapy, bone marrow taken from a matched donor is given to reconstitute the patient's (the host's) blood cells and immune system. The bone marrow has to be well matched so that the donor immune system cells will not recognize the host body tissue as foreign and mount an immune attack on it. In spite of an apparent match, sometimes there is an immediate and severe rejection reaction called acute graft versus host disease. This is treated with medication that suppresses the immune system and stops the rejection process.

In some cases there is a less severe form of rejection reaction that occurs over a period of months to years and consists of patches of thickened skin over the arms, legs, and trunk that is very similar to localized scleroderma. It is treated with some of the same medications that are used in acute graft versus host disease. The reaction can be controlled, but is seldom totally cured and therefore is termed chronic GVHD.

It should be noted that this reaction does not occur with kidney transplants, or other organ transplants since these organs do not contain immune cells. In the case of organ transplants the recipient's immune system is intact.

Eosinophilia Myalgia Syndrome (EMS)

Eosinophilia myalgia syndrome (EMS) was first described in 1989 and occurred in a group of patients who had taken a health food supplement with tryptophan that contained a contaminant, the nature of which is still uncertain. The health food supplement was taken off the market, and the "epidemic" subsided. However, there are still occasional cases that occur in people who have never taken any tryptophan supplements. The condition is characterized by thickened and tight skin over the extremities (usually sparing the hands and feet), swelling of the extremities, rash, and pain in muscles and joints. Muscle pain is a very prominent feature of this condition. Additionally, nerves can be affected, causing burning and stinging sensations in multiple areas of the body. Lung problems occur in about half of affected people.

IV

....

COPING
WITH
SCLERODERMA

16

* * *

YOU AND
YOUR DOCTOR

Prior to becoming ill, most people have little knowledge about the medical profession and all its subspecialties. Consequently, they may be unsure which type of doctor to go to about a specific problem.

In the early period, soon after getting diagnosed, scleroderma patients are frequently uncertain about what kind of doctor they should see, so they rely on the advice of their general medical doctor. This is precisely what they should do. Most patients will benefit from an evaluation by a specialist who knows scleroderma, and most of the time this will be a rheumatologist. Whether or not the rheumatologist provides ongoing care after this evaluation will vary from case to case.

The initial workup usually includes the following:

A comprehensive history and physical. The history includes information on your past medical problems, on your Raynaud's attacks, on difficulties (or lack of difficulties) with heartburn or trouble breathing, and a long list of other questions. The physical part is pretty basic, with a close examination of your skin, particularly your fingertips; listening to your lungs and heart with the stethoscope; evaluation of joint mobility, and so on. No part of this phase of the workup involves anything especially fancy, painful, complicated, or expensive.

Blood and urine tests. This will vary depending on what your primary doctor has done and on what the rheumatologist finds on the history and physical, but may include routine tests of blood counts, kidney, liver, and muscle function, as well as a test for the autoantibodies (antinuclear antibodies, or ANA) typically seen in the connective tissue diseases.

Baseline tests of internal organ involvement. It is impossible to give a list of tests that would apply to every scleroderma patient. Potentially this could include tests to evaluate the function of the lungs, heart, esophagus, stomach, and bowel. Which tests, if any, are done depend on what symptoms people have. In most circumstances I like to get baseline pulmonary function tests. These are tests that require a patient to breathe into a machine that measures lung volumes, airflow, and air exchange from the lungs into the blood. Not everyone needs this, however, particularly people who do a lot of exercise, who have very physically demanding jobs, or who tell me that they can still run seven-minute miles. The same is true of heart function and gastrointestinal problems. If these tests have been done in the recent past, I usually do not repeat them, but I want to see the actual reports that they are normal, not just the verbal report from the patient that another doctor said they were normal.

Specialized tests of internal organ involvement. If it is clear to me from the history and physical and/or from the baseline tests mentioned above that there is internal organ damage, the question then becomes how severe the damage is and whether it is progressive. In this case, special tests such as high-resolution CAT scans of the lungs, cardiac catheterization, or others may be necessary. This may require referral to other subspecialists.

Test after Test, Doctor after Doctor

My patients frequently express their frustration about having all these tests, each ordered, performed, and interpreted by a different doctor. They are confused as to the meaning of the results, and they worry that there is poor communication among their many physicians. Each doctor is prescribing something for one part of the body and seems to be uninterested in or, worse, less than knowledgeable about the whole process of scleroderma.

I wish I could offer an easy solution to this problem. The fact is that modern medicine is so complex that it is no longer possible for one physician to perform and interpret all the different tests (cardiac catheterization, stress tests, endoscopy, bronchoscopy, and others) and to know all the latest treatments for all the systems of the body. This is both good news and bad news. The good news is that today we can diagnose and treat hundreds of different conditions that could not be diagnosed accurately or treated effectively even a decade ago. The bad news is that you have to go to multiple doctors, undergo multiple tests (some "uncomfortable," which is the medical lingo for "painful"), and be confused by multiple and sometimes seemingly contradictory descriptions of what is wrong.

It is at this point that multiple doctors come into the picture and you, the patient, have to become actively involved in your care. The key issue is coordination of care and sharing of information. Medicine has become so complex that it is no longer possible for one doctor to provide all the services that are required by people with diseases that can affect multiple organs in various ways. Here is an opportunity to play an active role in your care and most doctors (and doctors' offices) will appreciate the contribution.

Tip number 1: Get copies of your own records and keep these in a file. It doesn't matter if you don't understand the terminology. You can read them if you like, but your role is really that of executive secretary. Do not rely on your doctor's office to send a copy. They say they will, and I am sure they mean it, but too many times the records are not sent, arrive too late, or are incomplete. Bring a copy with you, and do not give your only copy to the rheumatologist. Have the clerk make a copy on the spot and give you back your originals.

Tip number 2: Have the nurse put your records in your chart before the doctor sees you. It is time-saving for the physician to have the laboratory tests from a previous workup on the same day that he or she does the history and physical. I can often finalize my diagnosis and offer a plan of treatment if I have this information available on the same day I first see a patient. (Some people want a second opinion "fresh," that is, they do not want to bias the doctor based on previous opinions. That is okay, but be candid with your doctor about this. Even if you wish to do this, include copies of test results.)

Tip number 3: Identify the "quarterback." This is the doctor who is going to coordinate your care. This may be your general practitioner, your general internist, your rheumatologist, or another subspecialist. You have to be clear in your own mind, and it has to be made clear to your doctor, who is playing that role. For my scleroderma patients who need tests from other specialists, and who will likely get treatment based on the results of those tests, I want to be the one calling the shots.

When I send a patient to a pulmonologist (lung specialist) or other specialist, I want that doctor to do the evaluation and get back to me with the results before starting treatment. Usually when I refer a patient to them, I indicate that this is the arrangement. This is important to ensure that a medication from one doctor will not conflict with another or that a test recently done by one specialist will not be repeated by another.

Tip number 4: Make sure all your subspecialists have all the other doctors' reports. The best way to do this is to request a copy of each specialist's report to be sent to you directly. It is okay to do this, and people do it all the time. You are not meddling or being nosy. There is nothing secret in the reports. If you are afraid that there will be something in the report that will frighten you, don't read it. If you do read it and get alarmed, talk to your doctor about it. You can also ask the specialist to send a copy of the report to all your doctors. This does not involve much extra work on the doctor's part (the same letter gets sent), and the only added expense is the mailing cost. It is very helpful for you to have a typed list of the names and addresses of all your doctors, or a business card from all the doctors who are to get reports. Pick up a couple of extra cards when you go to a new doctor. In any event, make sure you get a copy of the report for your personal file. You may be referred to some new specialist in the future, and having your own copies would be helpful.

Keep in mind that all your body systems are interrelated. The results of the lung workup will be relevant to the heart doctor and the GI doctor. Sometimes they may only glance at them for a second and put them down again. Sometimes all they need to see is the bottom of the report, where it says "normal." It does not take much time to read this, but the information is extremely valuable.

Tip number 5: It is not necessary in most situations to have the specialist call your primary doctor. This kind of communication is usually done by letter, which is dictated on the same day that you are seen. The problem is not with making a phone call; the problem is with playing phone tag for days in a row.

Tip number 6: You and your primary care doctor are going to have a long-term relationship. Figure out who in the office is the person who handles referrals and is the one who can get the doctor's attention. This may be the office manager, the receptionist, or the nurse. Before you run into problems, find out when the best time is to call and when the doctor is likely to call back. Some doctors make return calls at lunch or in the evening. If you are having a problem, call as early in the day as possible.

Whom to Call

Let us assume that you get sick with something. You have at least four, sometimes five doctors (primary care physician, rheumatologist, pulmonologist, gastroenterologist, cardiologist) to choose from. This can be tricky, and the bottom line is that you have to make your own judgment call. If you really feel that the problem would be best addressed by, say, your rheumatologist but your insurance requires that you first contact your primary care physician, call the primary care person and ask immediately, over the phone, for a one-time extra referral. As you become more experienced with your condition, it will become easier and easier to make these decisions.

The Emergency Room

If you experience trouble breathing, chest pain, or high fevers, go to the emergency room (ER). If these problems start during the day, notify your doctor first. If you have a choice, go to the emergency room of the hospital where your doctor is on staff. In most other situations, avoid the ER. They do not understand scleroderma. You will spend at least four hours there, and they are likely to send you home with instructions to call your doctor.

In summary, your doctor wants to provide you with the best care in the most timely and cost-efficient manner. Likewise, you want to receive the best care, and you don't want to undergo tests over and over again because the prior test results are unavailable and your doctor can't proceed with treatment without knowing these results. On the other hand, you want to be sure that the proper tests are done so that problems can be identified early and treated as well as possible. This is going to take some effort on your part. Following the tips above and being an active participant in your own care will go a long way toward making sure that this happens. You and your doctor are partners in this endeavor.

17

* * *

LIVING AN
UNPREDICTABLE LIFE,
FACING AN
UNCERTAIN FUTURE

What is different about you the day *after* your disease was diagnosed from you the day *before*? For many people, what has changed is their sense of mortality, of vulnerability, of order in life—basically their sense of the future.

A diagnosis of a rare, chronic, incurable illness brings you up short. You are not in control, and it is this lack of control that is at the heart of the difficulty for many people. I try to point out to patients that in reality they have never been in control of much that happens inside their bodies, and indeed in their lives. In actuality, though, most of us live every day as if we *are* in control, and we plan for a future that *is* predictable on a day-to-day basis. It is not possible to live an organized and effective life without this attitude. We go to the grocery store and plan dinners for the coming week. We worry about paying the bills and taking care of aging parents. In terms of the long run, we make the assumption that we or our spouse will work until retirement, that we will get the kids through school, and that we will be taking a vacation next summer. Although we may have known people with serious illnesses that disrupted their life plans, they are not us. We usually feel that such illnesses aren't supposed to happen to us.

Suddenly all that predictability has changed. How can you continue to live an organized and effective life in the face of this uncertainty?

Living an Unpredictable Life

On hearing the diagnosis of scleroderma for the first time, people respond in different ways. Some people want to get as much information as possible right from the beginning, while others are content to go from visit to visit without giving much thought to the future. Most people want to know what they can expect from the disease. They want to know what is going to happen to them in the future. Most people also need time initially to summon the emotional strength to ask the "big" questions: "Will I die from this? Will I be disabled?" Sometimes these questions remain unasked, since people are afraid of the answers.

Although these are all simple and straightforward questions, the answers are not. Scleroderma has such a variable course from one person to the next that it is very difficult to predict what will happen to any individual patient. The course varies from mild disease in some cases to severe disease in others. Sometimes people who start out with very active and progressive disease reach a plateau and then slowly improve and do well in the long run.

There are some generalizations that can be made, however,

about the pace and course of disease activity. The skin thickening tends to reach its maximum point in the first two to five years. Then it usually reaches a stable stage and sometimes will improve even without treatment. The onset of internal organ involvement, on the other hand, is highly unpredictable. Lung and gastrointestinal involvement tends to happen within the first few years but can occur at any time. Over and over again, patients tell me that they developed a complication (such as kidney disease) ten years or more after the diagnosis and that their doctors had told them it was not supposed to happen after the first five years. For the most part, I no longer try to predict a patient's outcome. I treat the disease as it currently exists. I monitor tests for the development or worsening of internal organ involvement, and I treat problems as they arise.

Because of the differences among individual patients and even at different times in the same patient, I cannot give a straight answer to questions such as "How long will I be able to keep on working?" Many of my patients continue to work, but this depends to some extent on the type of job they hold. There *is* a future after the diagnosis. It simply may not be the one you had planned. It may be worse, but it in some ways it may be better. Perhaps I can best illustrate this with some stories concerning real patients.

One of my patients had a job at the airport collecting money for parking. She worked in a small outdoor booth and had to extend her hand out the window to every passing car. Although the booth was heated in the winter (and in Michigan the cold weather begins in September and ends in May), the window was usually open and she could not avoid cold exposure. This in-and-out exposure was disastrous for a scleroderma patient with Raynaud's phenomenon and a tendency to get recurrent finger ulcers. In her case, she did have to change her job.

Another of my patients is a piano teacher. The first doctor she saw told her to stop playing the piano, since it would cause too much pressure on her fingertips. She was devastated and became depressed. When I saw her, I realized that she had limited, mild scleroderma, and as long as she did not have an open ulcer on her finger, I saw no reason for her not to resume playing. The exercise was actually good for her hands. That was more than ten years ago. She and her husband are now retired, and she has voluntarily stopped teaching but still plays for her own enjoyment and that of her family.

Another of my patients, a young man, was a construction worker and, of course, was outdoors most of the time. He was unable to continue work due to intolerance to cold and to the clumsiness of his hands from the numbness that cold exposure caused—he said he could barely hold a hammer in the cold, much less use it well.

My oldest patient is currently ninety-three years old. She was diagnosed at the age of fifty. She sometimes uses a cane when she walks, to assist her balance, but gets around very well. She has outlived her husband and two of her doctors. Scleroderma has not interfered very much in her lifestyle over the past forty-three years, except she has had to make a few more adjustments to the cold more than she otherwise might have done.

Another one of my patients, a middle-aged man with a desk job for one of the car companies here in Detroit, told me the following story. At the height of his illness—and he had diffuse disease, with a lot of thick and tight skin on his hands, arms, face, trunk, and legs—his wife and daughter had to help him dress in the morning, especially to tie his shoes, since he could not bend over far enough to get his feet close to his hands, and he could not manipulate the laces to tie a tight bow. He said that one of his fears was that his shoes would become untied at work and he would be too embarrassed to ask a coworker to tie them for him. He continued to go to work every day, both on days when he felt good and on days when he felt awful. That was eight years ago. Over time and with medication, his skin softened and he regained a lot of his flexibility. Even though he was getting better, he decided to take early retirement (at age sixty) to spend more time with his family. He has not developed significant internal organ involvement. I don't see him in my office much anymore, since he is doing so well.

I have a patient who is a teacher in a middle school (sixth, seventh, and eighth grades). At the beginning of every school year she explains to her class why her hands look the way they do, why her fingers are so crooked. She lets them know that she will sometimes ask them for help with something she can't do. She tells me that she has no difficulty getting students to help out, but that still, after several years of explaining her situation to her students, it is tough every September.

My most complicated patient is a young woman with a twelve-year-old son and a devoted husband. Prior to her illness she was primarily a homemaker but had taught some aerobics classes and did some hair styling for extra income. Scleroderma was diagnosed five years ago. Now she is mostly bedridden. Her husband picks her up from bed to sit her up in the chair. She weighs less than 100 pounds. She can no longer walk because her knees do not straighten out. She can't comb her hair because she cannot raise her arm at the shoulder high enough to reach. Each day is a struggle for this family. There is no way I can paint a rosy picture of this situation. I marvel at their fortitude as I admire their courage.

Every patient's story is different. Some of these stories are happy; some are tragic. Often the stories are a combination of the two. Most of my patients do not see themselves as courageous or extraordinary in any way. Rather, they see themselves as coping the best they can with the choices available to them.

How individuals respond emotionally and psychologically to their condition is a reflection of their underlying personality and all the life experiences they have had up toward that point. People who have a tendency toward depression may become more depressed. People with a high degree of underlying anxiety will respond with greater nervousness and agitation. Some individuals, most commonly but not exclusively men, have difficulty dealing with feelings and may respond by becoming more distant and withdrawn. People with a strong sense of responsibility may see their illness as a failure to provide for their families.

All human beings resent sudden and undeserved loss. We all fear death and disability, and few of us are very enthusiastic about the unknown. There is no one "right" way to cope with your disease; you have to develop the way that suits you best.

The bookstores are filled with volumes on self-help and pop psychology. For the most part, these are uplifting and helpful. But there are some popular myths that may get in the way of your ability to come to terms with this new level of unpredictability in life and with the new identity that it brings. The following are several popular myths that I think are particularly harmful.

Myth number 1: You are in control of your body; whether you have mild disease or severe disease depends on how you respond to it.

Response: Whether you have mild disease or severe disease depends on your genetic predisposition to the disease and the level of the "triggering" factor (whatever the cause) you were exposed to. No amount of positive thinking will make scleroderma magically disappear. However, you may have more control than you realize over how you are affected by the disease. In this case, the key point is to appreciate the difference between pain and suffering.

Pain is the physiological response to a harmful stimulus. This is necessary for survival to make sure that individuals avoid injury. Suffering, on the other hand, is the emotional and psychological response to pain or any unpleasant situation. Pain is always worse at night, when there are no distractions to keep our minds off the problem and when fatigue is added to the sensation of pain. The extent to which pain bothers us depends on what else is going on. A paper cut can be a mild annoyance if we are engaged in a really exciting activity, such as watching a favorite sports team win a very close match, or it can be a major discomfort if we are preparing our taxes and it is April 15. Perhaps the worst suffering is experienced not even by the person having the pain, but by a loved one who feels he or she can only stand by helplessly and watch.

Suffering is made worse by many things. Anxiety over not knowing where the pain is coming from can turn an episode of heartburn into an imaginary heart attack. Becoming more informed about your condition is a good way to deal with this type of anxiety. Although you may not like what the answer is, at least you will know the facts. I frequently see patients who are referred for the purpose of confirming the diagnosis of scleroderma. Even when I tell them that the suspicion of their doctor is correct and that they do, in fact, have scleroderma, they frequently express a sense of relief, since now they have a name for their condition, a reason that they are having all these strange symptoms, and an approach to treatment that makes sense. Fear of the unknown is almost always worse than knowing the true situation.

For some people, the most important source of suffering is the fear of loss—loss of function if the hands are involved, loss of importance if livelihood is interrupted, loss of identity as homemaker or breadwinner, loss of physical attractiveness. How do you get in control of this fear?

The key issue is one of identity. Identity changes throughout life, but most of the time these changes are gradual and fairly predictable. Having survived the great adolescent identity crisis, most people are still shocked at the change in their identity after the birth of their first child. Middle age happens very gradually and should come as a surprise to no one, but nonetheless gray hairs and wrinkles are seldom welcome. Retirement is a huge emotional transition for many people, even though it is quite predictable. Developing scleroderma also brings an identity crisis, made worse by its totally unexpected occurrence and by its complete unfamiliarity. A diagnosis makes many people feel as if they have changed from Jane Doe, teacher and mother of two, to Jane Doe, scleroderma patient.

The first step in handling the situation, and thereby regaining emotional equilibrium, is to accept the idea that a change in identity, that is, a change in self-perception, is occurring. There is a "new you," and like the previous new yous of grown-up or parent or retiree, this transition is a process that occurs over an extended period of time. You also don't become a new you in a vacuum; your change in self-perception is influenced by your loved ones—spouse, children, friends. Unless they are brought along in this process, they will continue to expect the old you. You will probably need help in convincing them that the old you isn't around anymore. They may desperately want the old you to remain because they too are afraid of the unknown. There is frequently resentment over the fact that although *you* have the disease, *they* have to make changes. But people who really love you *will* change. Open communication, perhaps with the help of a family counselor, priest, minister, or rabbi, can make all the difference in the world.

Myth number 2: All life experiences are an opportunity for growth.

Response: Getting a diagnosis of a chronic, possibly debilitating disease is not good news, and no matter how your rephrase it, it is very difficult to see it as an opportunity. A true opportunity is one that, if you had to live your life over, you would freely choose again, although the benefits may not have been apparent at the time. An example of this tragedy-turned-opportunity is most often seen in individuals who have lost their job and who then go through a difficult time of reassessment, discover their true calling, and end up much more satisfied than if they had remained in their original, secure, but unfulfilling occupation. I have never had a scleroderma patient, even those who do quite well, describe their situation as a true opportunity. The fact is that some life experiences are bad, and personal growth can be very painful.

However, I have had many patients tell me how scleroderma forced them to reevaluate their lives and their priorities. Rather than being caught up on the treadmill of jobs and responsibilities, they stepped back and decided what was truly important. This is almost always family and relationships. They become aware that their most precious gift is time spent with loved ones.

Family members and loved ones have to be let in, not kept out. Isolation is damaging to the patient and devastating to any relationship. Family counseling may be necessary to assist in this process. Family members may feel lost and abandoned and just as out of control of the situation as the patient. Having a neutral person with whom to discuss these feelings and a safe environment in which to bring them up are important parts of keeping open the lines of communication.

As strange as it may sound, some relationships deepen and are strengthened by dealing with this adversity. I want to emphasize that I am not asking you to be happy about having scleroderma; rather, I am suggesting that you can use this to develop a better understanding of yourself and a deeper relationship with your loved ones.

The Difference between "Suffering From" and "Living With"

There is a difference between being a victim suffering from a disease and being a person living with a condition. The difference is more than just attitude. The term *victim* is fraught with a sense of passivity and helplessness. It brings to mind individuals whose lives were overrun by forces so much more powerful than they that they had no hope of influencing their own fate. On the other hand, the term *person living with . . .* implies an individual identity influenced but not overwhelmed by the condition. It combines a sense of acceptance of the condition (after all, there is no choice) with the notion that the person has an identity other than that defined by the disease. It should be clear that I prefer the second designation. The point is that although the disease may change your self-perception, it does not have to dominate your existence.

Myth number 3: We all face an uncertain future; your situation is no different from that of anyone else.

Response: The weather is uncertain, but the fact that the sun will come up tomorrow is considered a sure bet. Human beings get used to a particular level of certainty, which permits them to structure their lives accordingly. A diagnosis of an incurable disease, especially one with an uncertain prognosis or outcome, introduces a level of uncertainty that is above and beyond the usual level future and does indeed represent a new reality. People get used to a greater level of uncertainty.

In my practice I have noticed that people with a new diagnosis of scleroderma have a great many questions in the beginning. I can answer the trivial ones ("Why am I stiff? Why do I have heartburn?"), but I cannot answer the important ones ("What causes scleroderma? What is the cure?"). After a while, people have fewer questions as they become more familiar with and more knowledgeable about their own condition.

Where to Get Help

The Scleroderma Foundation has chapters and support groups around the country. Appendix 2 lists the foundation's contact information as well as other organizations that provide support and information.

✳   ✳   ✳

This book ends with a view to the future. We now know more about scleroderma than ever before. Research continues daily, and progress, though slow, is being made. New treatments are being developed to better deal with symptoms, prevent progression, and improve well-being. One day the cause will be known and the cure will be found.

Appendix 1
❋ ❋ ❋

American College of Rheumatology

CRITERIA FOR THE CLASSIFICATION OF SYSTEMIC SCLERODERMA

Major Criterion:

Skin thickness of the fingers plus skin thickness extending over the back of the hand.

Minor Criteria:

1. Skin thickness of the fingers (sclerodactyly)
2. Pulmonary fibrosis in the bases of the lungs
3. Digital pitting scars, ulcers, or loss of finger pad substance

A diagnosis of scleroderma is considered definite if either the single major criterion is present, or if at least two of the three minor criteria are present.

Localized forms of scleroderma and sclerodermalike disorders are excluded from these criteria.

Adapted from A. T. Masi, G. P. Rodnan, T. A. Medsger Jr., et al., Preliminary criteria for the classification of systemic sclerosis (scleroderma). *Arthritis and Rheumatism* 23(1980): 581-90.

Appendix 2

✳ ✳ ✳

SCLERODERMA SUPPORT GROUPS AND RESOURCE MATERIAL

U.S. Patient support and information

Arthritis Foundation
National office: 1314 Spring St., NW
Atlanta, GA 30309
Telephone: 404-872-7100 or 800-283-7800
    The Arthritis Foundation has local chapters throughout the United States and has literature on all the connective tissue diseases, including scleroderma. The Arthritis Foundation raises funds for research on all these diseases.

Scleroderma Foundation
89 Newbury Street, Suite 210
Danvers, MA 01923
Telephone: 800-722-4673 or 978-750-4499
Fax: 978-750-9902
E-mail: sclerofed@aol.com
World Wide Web address: http://www.scleroderma.com
    The Scleroderma Foundation has local chapters and support groups throughout the United States and has affiliated groups in Canada. The foundation raises funds for research, publishes literature

on scleroderma, sponsors conferences, and conducts public aware-
ness campaigns.

Scleroderma Research Foundation
2320 Bath Street, Suite 315
Santa Barbara, CA 93105
Telephone: 805-563-9133 or 800-441-CURE
World Wide Web address: http://www.srfcure.org
    This foundation also raises funds to support research.

National Institutes of Health
1 AMS Circle
Bethesda, MD 20892-3675
Telephone: 301-495-4484
Fax: 301-718-6366
World Wide Web address: http://www.nih.gov/niams/
    National Arthritis and Musculoskeletal and Skin Diseases Infor-
mation Clearinghouse, a public service sponsored by the National
Institute of Arthritis and Musculoskeletal and Skin Diseases (NIAMS)
of the National Institutes of Health (NIH). The Clearinghouse distrib-
utes National Institute of Arthritis and Musculoskeletal and Skin Dis-
eases publications; it also maintains a file in the Combined Health
Information Database (CHID), publicly accessible on the Internet.
Materials indexed in CHID include books, pamphlets, journal arti-
cles, and audiovisuals. Personal information requests are fulfilled by
Information Specialists and referred to other appropriate organizations for additional information.

Outside the United States

Raynaud's and Scleroderma Association
112 Crewe Road
Alsager, Cheshire ST7 2JA
England
Telephone: 01270 872776
Fax: 01270 883556
E-mail: webmaster@raynauds.demon.co.uk
World Wide Web address: http://www.raynauds.demon.co.uk

Associazione Patologie Autoimmuni
Via degli Uliveti, 8
Silvi Marina
64029 Teremo Italy
Phone: 011 39 085.935.35.60

Books and Pamphlets on Scleroderma Written for Patients

The following three books are all available from the Scleroderma Foundation (address listed above).

Mark Flapan, *Perspectives on Living with Scleroderma*. Scleroderma Federation, 1997.

E. Carwile LeRoy, M.D., *Understanding and Managing Scleroderma*. Scleroderma Federation, 1996.

Dana Lovvorn, *Scleroderma: Surviving the Seventeen Year Itch*. United Scleroderma Foundation, 1996.

Literature on Scleroderma for Doctors

Philip J. Clements and Daniel E. Furst, eds., *Systemic Sclerosis*. Williams and Wilkins, 1996.

V. D. Steen, ed., "Scleroderma—Preface," introduction to a special issue on scleroderma, *Rheumatic Disease Clinics of North America*, vol. 22, no. 4, 1996.

Carol M. Black and Allen R. Myers, eds., *Systemic Sclerosis (Scleroderma)*. Gower Medical Publishing, 1985.

General Rheumatology Textbooks

William N. Kelly, et al., *Textbook of Rheumatology*, 4th ed. W. B. Saunders, 1996.

John H. Klippel and Paul A. Dieppe, *Rheumatology*, 2nd ed. Mosby, 1997.

Daniel J. McCarty and William J. Koopman, *Arthritis and Allied Conditions: A Textbook of Rheumatology*. Lea and Febiger, 1993.

Glossary

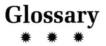

Aldolase: a muscle enzyme normally present in low levels in the blood, but elevated to high levels in conditions like polymyositis in which there is muscle destruction

Alveolitis: inflammation of the small air sacs in the lungs

Alveolus, pl. *alveoli*: small air sac in the lung

American College of Rheumatology (ACR): the professional organization of rheumatologists

Anemia: low number of red cells and/or low amount of hemoglobin in the blood

Antibody: a protein made by cells of the immune system that attacks a substance, usually a foreign substance, in the body

Anticentromere antibody: an antibody directed against a protein in the cell nucleus; it is found most often in patients with limited scleroderma but can be seen occasionally in other conditions

Anti-DNA antibody: an antibody directed against genetic material in the cell; it is usually seen in lupus patients and only rarely seen in scleroderma patients

Antinuclear antibody: an antibody directed against one of the many components in the nucleus (internal compartment containing the genes) of the cell

Antitopoisomerase antibody: an antibody directed against an enzyme in the nucleus; it is also called the Scl-70 antibody and is seen in about 25 percent of scleroderma patients, usually those with diffuse skin involvement

Arrhythmia: abnormal heart rhythm

Arthralgia: pain in the joints

Arthritis: inflammation in the joints

Atrial fibrillation: a form of abnormal heart rhythm in which the heart beats in an irregular pattern

Autoantibody: a protein made by cells of the immune system that attacks the body's own tissues

Autoimmune disease: a disease in which the immune system attacks the body's own tissue, also called connective tissue disease; the most common autoimmune diseases are rheumatoid arthritis, lupus, scleroderma, polymyositis, and Sjogren's syndrome

Autonomic nervous system: that part of the nervous system that controls the inner workings of the body; it is divided into the sympathetic and parasympathetic systems

Barrette's esophagus: a precancerous change in the lining cells of the esophagus at the area near the stomach

Bell's palsy: weakness or paralysis of the muscles on one side of the face; also called seventh nerve palsy; a form of cranial neuropathy

Biopsy: the process of taking a small piece of tissue to examine under the microscope

Bradycardia: abnormally slow heart rhythm; also called *brady-arrhythmia*

Broncho-alveolar lavage: a procedure in which liquid is first introduced into one area of the lungs (through a bronchoscope) and then suctioned out to get samples of mucus to determine whether there is infection, inflammation, or cancer

Bronchoscopy: a procedure in which a tube is passed into the lungs

Bronchus, pl. *bronchi*: large air tube in the lung

BUN: Blood urea nitrogen, a substance in the blood that is one of the breakdown products of the body; it is normally excreted by the kidneys, so a high BUN suggests that the kidneys are not functioning well

Calcinosis: calcium deposits in the skin or just below the skin, commonly seen in scleroderma, but also occurring in some other diseases

Calcium channel blocker: a type of medication that results in opening up (dilatation) of the blood vessels, used to improve circulation, to lower blood pressure, or to treat some types of heart disease

Capillary: the smallest blood vessel in the body

Cardiology: the branch of medicine that treats heart disease

Carpal tunnel syndrome: numbness and tingling of the hand due to pressure on the median nerve at the wrist; this is one form of compression neuropathy

Collagen: a fibrous protein made by cells that provides the firmness in the skin, forms the lining of organs, and is the basic structural protein in bones, tendons, ligaments, and joints

Colonoscopy: a procedure of passing a tube into the colon

Connective tissue diseases: autoimmune diseases including rheumatoid arthritis, lupus, scleroderma, polymyositis, and Sjogren's syndrome

Constriction: narrowing

Contracture: bending of a joint, the inability to fully straighten out a joint

Cortisone: a powerful antiinflammatory medication that occurs naturally, at low levels, in the body; a type of steroid

CPK: Creatine phosphokinase, a muscle enzyme, the blood level of which is elevated when muscle is damaged, for example, with heart muscle damage in a heart attack or with skeletal muscle damage in myositis

Cranial neuropathy: disease of one of the cranial nerves that provide sensation and muscle movement to the face and head

Creatinine: a substance in the blood that is abnormally high when the kidneys do not work normally

CREST: an acronym that stands for calcinosis, Raynaud's phenomenon, esophageal dysfunction, sclerodactyly, and telangiectasia; describes a form of scleroderma

Dermatology: the branch of medicine that treats skin diseases

Dermatomyositis: a disease with inflammation of the muscles, causing weakness, and inflammation of the skin, causing a rash

Dermis: the skin

Dialysis: use of a machine that cleanses the blood of waste products when the kidneys are unable to do so

Digital pits: tiny, indented areas in the fingertips that are typical of scleroderma

Digital ulcers: open sores on the fingers or toes

Digits: fingers and toes

Dilate: to open up

DLCO: diffusion in liters of carbon monoxide; a test that measures the ability of the lungs to get oxygen into the blood

Duodenum: the first part of the bowel after the stomach

Dysphagia: difficulty swallowing

Dyspnea: shortness of breath

Echocardiogram: an ultrasound test of the heart

Edema: swelling

Edematous: swollen

Endocrinology: the branch of medicine that treats diseases of the glands, such as thyroid disease and diabetes

Endoscopy: a procedure that involves passing a tube into the esophagus and stomach (upper endoscopy) or into the colon (lower endoscopy or colonoscopy)

Entrapment neuropathy: damage to a nerve due to pressure along its course; also known as compression neuropathy

Eosinophilia myalgia syndrome (EMS): a condition characterized by muscle pain and inflammation, nerve inflammation, and increased eosinophils in the blood

Eosinophilic fasciitis: a sclerodermalike illness that has inflammation in the area just beneath the skin and fat, called the fascia

Eosinophils: one of the types of white blood cells; they are increased in some cases of scleroderma and in some of the sclerodermalike disorders

Epidermis: the outermost layer of the skin, specially adapted to provide protection against most injuries. Injury limited to the epidermis does not result in a scar. Examples of this are sunburns and shallow scratches. Scleroderma is primarily a disease of the dermis, the lower layer of skin beneath the epidermis

Esophagitis: inflammation of the lining of the esophagus

Esophagus: the swallowing tube between the mouth and the stomach

Fasciitis: inflammation of the fascia, a layer that separates muscles from the overlying fat and skin

Fibroblast: a cell that makes collagen

Fibrosis: scar tissue buildup that replaces normal tissue

Gastritis: inflammation of the lining of the stomach

Gastroenterology: the branch of medicine that deals with digestive and liver problems

Gastroesophageal reflux disease (GERD): a condition in which stomach acid passes up into the esophagus, usually causing heartburn and damage to the lining of the esophagus

Gastroesophageal stricture: a narrowing of the junction between the esophagus and the stomach, usually as a result of recurrent acid reflux, which causes scar tissue buildup

Gastrointestinal tract (GI tract): the digestive system, including the esophagus, stomach, duodenum, small bowel, large bowel or colon, and rectum; it also includes the liver and gall bladder

Graves' disease: a thyroid condition usually characterized by an overactive thyroid gland

H-2 blocker: a type of medicine that decreases acid secretion in the stomach

Hashimoto's disease or *Hashimoto's thyroiditis*: a thyroid disease that usually results in an underactive thyroid

Heart block: a defect in the electrical system of the heart that can cause an abnormal pulse

HLA test: histocompatibility locus antigens test, a blood test to determine the genes that control the immune system; usually only done for research

Holter monitor: a portable instrument that measures heartbeat for an extended period of time (usually twenty-four hours) to detect abnormalities in the heart rate that occur intermittently

Hyperpigmentation: too much pigment, or darker-than-normal skin

Hypopigmentation: loss of pigment, or lighter-than-normal skin

Infarction: death of tissue from lack of blood supply

Ischemia: lowered blood supply

Leucopenia: abnormally low white blood cell count

Linear scleroderma: a form of localized scleroderma in which the thickened skin is in the pattern of a line on the face or down an arm or leg

Lupus or *systemic lupus erythematosus (SLE)*: an autoimmune disease characterized by inflammation in multiple organ systems, frequently involving skin, joints, and the kidneys

Lymphopenia: abnormally low lymphocyte count

Malabsorption: decreased absorption of nutrients in the bowel; in scleroderma this is due to decreased bowel motility and overgrowth of bacteria, resulting in diarrhea and weight loss

Malignant phase hypertension: a sudden and dangerous increase in blood pressure that can result in kidney failure if not treated

MCTD: mixed connective tissue disease, a disease characterized by features of lupus, scleroderma, and polymyositis, usually with a positive anti-RNP antibody test

Morphea: a form of localized scleroderma characterized by patches of thickened skin

Myocardial infarction (MI): heart attack

Myocarditis: inflammation of the heart muscle

Myositis: muscle inflammation

Neuralgia: pain of the nerve

Neuropathy: damage to nerves

Neuritis: inflammation of nerves

Nonsteroidal antiinflammatory drugs (NSAIDs): a class of medication that inhibits inflammation by decreasing prostaglandins

Osteoarthritis: a wear-and-tear arthritis, or degenerative arthritis, that occurs with age

Osteoporosis: thinning of bones due to loss of calcium

Pacemaker: a device that controls heart rhythm

Parasympathetic nervous system: part of the autonomic nervous system that controls the functioning of the internal organs

Pericarditis: inflammation of the sac that surrounds the heart

Pericardium: the sac that surrounds the heart

Peristalsis: the normal motility, or muscle activity, in the esophagus, stomach, and bowel

Pigmentation: skin color

Pleurisy: inflammation of the lining of the lungs, usually painful

Polymyositis: inflammation of the muscles

Prednisone: a form of cortisone or steroid hormone that is a powerful anti-inflammatory medication

Primary biliary cirrhosis (PBC): scarring in the liver caused by damage to the small bile ducts, seen occasionally in scleroderma and not related to alcohol

Prokinetic agent: a medication that improves motility

Proteinuria: protein in the urine

Proton pump inhibitor: a medication that decreases stomach acid

Pruritis: itching

Pulmonary fibrosis: scar tissue buildup in the lungs that interferes with normal function

Pulmonary function tests: tests performed by blowing into an instrument that measures lung volume, airflow, and ability to get oxygen into the blood

Pulmonary hypertension: high blood pressure in the pulmonary arteries; this can occur in the absence of high blood pressure as measured in the arm

Pulmonology: the branch of medicine that treats lung diseases

Raynaud's phenomenon: color changes of the fingers on cold exposure, usually white, then blue, then red; if it occurs alone it is called primary Raynaud's disease; if it occurs with scleroderma or lupus, it is called secondary Raynaud's phenomenon

Reflux: usually referring to gastroesophageal reflux, the backflow of acid from the stomach into the esophagus

Rheumatoid arthritis: an inflammatory autoimmune arthritis of multiple joints characterized by joint deformity and destruction

Rheumatology: the branch of medicine that treats all forms of arthritis and the autoimmune diseases

Sclerodactyly: thickening of the skin of the fingers

Sclerosis: hardening

Scl-70: an autoantibody in the blood that occurs in about 25 percent of scleroderma patients and usually is found in those with diffuse skin disease; also known as antitopoisomerase antibody

SLE: systemic lupus erythematosus (see *lupus*)

Steroid: a class of hormone that is either anti-inflammatory (gluco-corticoids, cortisone, prednisone) or one of the sex hormones (estrogen or testosterone)

Stricture: narrowing

Subcutaneous: under the skin

Sympathetic nervous system: part of the autonomic nervous system that controls the function of internal organs

Telangiectasias: small red spots on the skin due to enlargement of tiny blood vessels

Tendonitis: inflammation of tendons

Tendon rub: a sound like rubbing two pieces of leather together, made by the motion of a tendon in an inflamed tendon sheath; it is characteristic of scleroderma but can also occur after injury to a tendon

Thrombocytopenia: abnormally low platelets

Thrombocytosis: abnormally high platelets

Total parenteral nutrition (TPN): a form of feeding through veins for individuals who cannot maintain nutrition by eating

Watermelon stomach: a striped appearance of the lining of the stomach due to thinning of the mucous layer and dilatation of the underlying blood vessels; it frequently is associated with bleeding from these blood vessels

Index

✳ ✳ ✳